ON CALL IN
ANESTHESIA
AND SURGERY

D0108020

On Call in Anesthesia and Surgery

Ronald A. Malt, M.D.

Professor of Surgery
Harvard Medical School
Massachusetts General Hospital
Boston, Massachusetts

Gilles Chemtob, M.D.

Department of Anaesthesia
Royal Victoria Hospital
Montreal, Quebec
Canada

W.B. SAUNDERS COMPANY

A Division of Harcourt Brace & Company
Philadelphia London Toronto Montreal Sidney Tokyo

W.B. SAUNDERS COMPANY
A Division of Harcourt Brace & Company
The Curtis Center
Independence Square West
Philadelphia, PA 19106

Library of Congress Catalog Number 94-68177

ON CALL IN ANESTHESIA AND SURGERY   0-7216-3884-8

Printed in the United States of America

Last digit is the print number: 9   8   7   6   5   4   3   2   1

PREFACE

No one works closer, in all respects, than do residents in surgery and in anesthesia. Nevertheless, the flow of reciprocal information is frequently suboptimal.

For these reasons, in 1987, Drs. J. Bucknam McPeek, Michael Bailin, Paul Alfille, and others enthusiastically accepted the challenge to represent the educational interests of anesthetists, while Henry Mankin and I stood up for surgery, helped by Drs. P.K. Donahoe (pediatric surgery), R.B. Donoff and J. Wilkes (maxillofacial surgery), S.P. Dretler (urology), D. Mathisen (thoracic surgery), J.W. May (plastic surgery), R.L. Fabian (eye, ear, nose, and throat), G.S. Richardson (obstetrics and gynecology), and N.T. Zervas (neurosurgery). We resolved to develop a handbook useful for trainees in our disciplines, perhaps with carryover elsewhere.

Despite initial enthusiasm, of course, none of us actually had as much time to set forth our precepts and biases as we would have liked.

Activity slowed, then stopped. We were unhappy. Fortunately, in April, 1991, Mike Bailin identified Gilles Chemtob, a former fellow in critical care medicine at Massachusetts General Hospital, now on the attending staff at the Royal Victoria Hospital, McGill University, in Montreal, as someone who might shoulder a major part of the scholarly burden in helping to meld the disparate requirements of the surgical and anesthesia residents.

Although the handbook was originally *Surgery for Anesthetists*, it nearly became *Anesthesiology for Surgeons:* just the kind of reciprocity we all wanted and, moreover, a *vade mecum* for residents in both anesthesiology and surgery facing their board examinations.

As matters developed further, however, we and our residents discerned that the handbook, whatever it was to be called, was a lifeline to residents without a more experienced staff member at hand.

November, 1993
Ronald A. Malt, M.D., Boston
Gilles Chemtob, M.D., C.M., Montreal

DESCRIPTION OF LAYOUT

Following is an explanation of the layout of the surgical procedures described in this book:

SURGICAL PROCEDURE

Conventional name plus additional pertinent comments.

Objective   Surgical goals of the procedure.

Position   Patient's position intraoperatively.

Exposure   Area of body that is prepped and draped.

Incision   Surgical incision necessary for procedure.

Blood Bank Order   Recommended blood bank orders; will vary in different institutions.

Estimated Blood Loss   Depends on method of measuring blood loss, the surgeon's skill, the patient population, and the anesthetic management.

Preoperative Studies   Listed for each surgical procedure is the recommended preoperative laboratory studies for the administration of that anesthetic. "Routine" implies the minimum recommended laboratory data in an otherwise healthy patient without any associated medical abnormalities. The following minimum recommended laboratory data will vary in different institutions.
Children Hb
Adult
<40 y: women, Hb; men, none.
>40 and <60 y: women and men, Hb, BUN, creatinine, glucose, electrolytes, ECG
>60 y: women and men, Hb, creatinine, BUN, glucose, electrolytes, ECG; CXR optional

Anesthetic Choices   The anesthetic technique(s) feasible for the procedure. However, one may always consider the following options:
1. No anesthesia, i.e., anesthesia personnel not needed or the anesthesiologist declines to administer an anesthetic because the patient's condition has not been optimized.
2. Local with or without IV sedation: monitored anesthesia care
3. Regional technique: major nerve blocks, e.g., spinal
4. General anesthesia: mask or intubated
5. Combined technique: general anesthesia plus regional anesthesia

Invasive Monitoring   Refers to invasive monitoring recommended over and above routine monitoring. Routine monitoring should consist of the standards as recommended by the American Society of Anesthesiologists (ASA) (described in the back of the member's guide) or the Canadian Anesthesiologists' Society's (CAS) guidelines (described in March 1993 supplement). Routine monitoring consists of the following:
1. Continuous anesthesia: personnel present
2. Continuous monitoring of:
   a. Oxygenation (Sao_2, Fio_2 analyzer, a visible body part)
   b. Ventilation ($ETCO_2$ for intubated patient is standard monitoring as recommended by CAS; disconnect alarm; respirator)
   c. Circulation (ECG, BP, other, e.g., stethoscope or arterial line)
3. Availability of temperature monitoring equipment
4. Other recommended but not essential equipment: anesthetic gas concentration monitor, nerve stimulator.

Airway Considerations   Refers to whether special precautions or considerations must be taken with regard to the airway management.

Aspiration Considerations   Refers to whether or when patients should have "full stomach" considerations.

Estimated Surgical Time   Approximate average duration of procedure. Variability depends on surgeon and patient.

➤ **Anesthetic Considerations**
All anesthetic considerations considered important.

Intraoperative Hazards   Particular or important dangers, whether related to surgery or to anesthesia.

Postoperative Pain Control   Measures commonly used to control postoperative pain. Routine measures refers to IM route (e.g., narcotics—meperidine 1 mg/kg q1–4h prn or ketorolac 10–30 mg q4–6h; maximum 120 mg/d) or PO analgesic (e.g., codeine, acetaminophen, or other nonsteroidal antiinflammatory drug [NSAID]).

APPENDIX I

Common Surgical Positions   Illustrations of the seven most common surgical positions.

APPENDIX II

Commonly Used Medical Abbreviations   The abbreviations used in the text.

CONTENTS

CHAPTER 1

CARDIOVASCULAR PROCEDURES

Aortic Procedures

SURGICAL PROCEDURE Abdominal Aortic Surgery

1. Abdominal aortic aneurysms (AAA) are classified by location (infrarenal or suprarenal) and by size. Usually 5 cm is considered the size of potential bursting. LaPlace's law holds.
2. They occur most commonly in elderly men.
3. Most patients are atherosclerotic; therefore systemic atherosclerosis and coronary artery disease (CAD) are concerns.

Objective Excision of abdominal aneurysm; replacement with graft.

Position Supine; or tilted to the right or left for retroperitoneal approaches.

Exposure Nipples to knees.

Incision Midline transabdominal; or right or left retroperitoneal oblique.

Blood Bank Order Type and crossmatch (T&C) 4–6 units PRBC; if aneurysm has ruptured, T&C 10 units PRBC; autotransfusion techniques useful: predonation, intraoperative hemodilution, intraoperative blood salvage. Consider use of antifibrinolytics (e.g., tranexamic acid, aprotinin).

Predonation Guidelines If Hb > 11 g/dl, autologous blood can be donated every 3 days up to 5 weeks before surgery—longer if blood is stored frozen.

Estimated Blood Loss 500 to 1000 ml.

Preoperative Studies CBC, coagulation profile, electrolytes, BUN, creatinine, glucose, LFTs, CXR, ECG.
    Comments: Further cardiac, pulmonary, and cerebrovascular workup often required in terms of consults and laboratory studies.

Anesthetic Choices General anesthesia or combined general and regional anesthesia.
    Comments: Combined technique is most common. Thoracic or lumbar epidural catheter or spinal catheter is placed preoperatively because the

1

potential for postoperative coagulopathy prohibits postoperative place-ment. A thoracic epidural catheter is technically more difficult to place than a lumbar catheter is and may carry slightly higher risks.

Invasive Monitoring   Arterial line, Foley, central venous catheter (CVC); pul-monary artery catheter (PAC) and transesophageal echocardiography (TEE) optional.

Comments: PAC is not necessarily placed. Depends on patient's under-lying medical problems. In patients with good ventricular function with-out significant valvular disease or pulmonary hypertension, one can do with just a CVC. Recommend sheath introducer as a CVC. It can serve as a large-bore IV access and to facilitate insertion of a PAC if it should become indicated during the procedure. TEE is useful during abdominal aortic surgery for assessment of cardiac function, ischemia, and fluids primarily.

Aspiration Precautions   Not necessary unless an emergency procedure (e.g., leaking, expanding, or ruptured aneurysms) or patient is at risk of gastric reflux.

Queries for Surgeon   Infrarenal or suprarenal aneurysm? Affects extent of renal protective measures required.

➤ **Anesthetic Considerations**
  1. **Anesthetic Goals**
     a. Evaluate and optimize patient preoperatively (e.g., uncontrolled hy-pertension or prerenal failure).
     b. Maintain stable hemodynamics despite changes in stimulation and loading conditions. Provide smooth induction. Replace extensive 3rd space fluid losses (approximately 10–15 ml/kg/h) and blood loss (3:1 crystalloid replacement to blood loss). Control and reduce BP before aortic cross-clamping. Replenish circulating volume. Moderately ele-vate BP and preload before cross-clamp is removed. Provide adequate analgesia on emergence from anesthesia and after surgery.
     c. Protect and closely monitor major organs at risk: heart (cardiac isch-emia, failure, and arrhythmias), kidneys (renal failure; approximately 40% decreased renal blood flow with infrarenal clamp), lungs (pul-monary complications).
  2. **Preoperative Evaluation**
     Pay special attention to generalized atherosclerosis, CAD, cerebrovascular disease (N.B.: asymptomatic carotid bruit does not need further workup), renovascular disease, history of smoking and pulmonary disease, diabetes mellitus.
  3. **Preoperative Medications**
     On the morning of surgery, patient receives usual cardiac and antihy-pertensive medication and morphine (0.1 mg/kg) IM, plus a benzodiaze-pine to relieve anxiety if necessary. Antacids (H_2-receptor blockers) are useful in the obese and in patients with esophageal reflux or who are difficult to intubate. Two cimetidine pills will normally do.
  4. **Setup & Monitoring**
     Usual anesthetic setup plus large-bore IV access connected to a blood administration set and fluid warmer; warming blanket; temperature mon-itoring; prewarm OR and blankets to cover patient during induction; CVC

sheath (introducer) with or without PAC set, epidural set, IV drips (vasopressors, vasodilators, and dopamine for renal protection), NG tube, autotransfuser.

Comments: PAC is not always necessary but is useful in patient with suspected or known cardiac dysfunction or hemodynamic compromise.

5. **Intraoperative Management**

Usual patient identification; monitoring placed on patient: leads II and V_5 monitored simultaneously; large-bore IV access; proper placement of epidural tested before induction; conventional induction with special cardiac considerations (smooth, controlled induction); CVC with or without PAC can be placed after induction; ETT, NGT, and Foley placement. Monitor depth of paralysis with twitch monitor. Ensure that patient has received surgical antibiotic prophylaxis. Before cross-clamping is done, ensure

a. Renal protection (mannitol, furosemide, and dopamine drips if indicated)
b. Control of BP in low normal range
c. Heparinization 5000–7000 units IV.

Note time and duration of cross-clamping. Limit aortic cross-clamping time to <2 hours to prevent lower extremity ischemia (rhabdomyolysis and compartment syndromes). Before cross-clamping is removed, ensure circulating volume is replenished and BP elevated. Protamine reversal is done after clamp is removed. Verify activated clotting time (ACT). Patients may be extubated immediately after surgery in routine, uncomplicated elective procedures when patient has no appreciable hypothermia, is hemodynamically stable, and has no severe underlying disease.

6. **Intraoperative Management of Ruptured AAA**

Goal: Surgical access to aorta for cross-clamping. If patient has rapidly deteriorating BP or even has no detectable BP, call for additional help; ABCs (airway, breathing, and circulation) provided as for any resuscitation (including oxygen, ventilation, and intubation); IV access (large bore) obtained and paralysis provided as soon as possible while patient is prepped and draped and abdomen is incised by surgeon. Massive fluid resuscitation. Administer blood (type O negative if crossmatch not available); insert radial cutdown and CVC. As patient stabilizes, attend to routine tasks: Give incremental doses of anesthetic; get blood for laboratory studies; review available chart.

Intraoperative Hazards

1. Specific surgical hazards:
   a. Expanding, leaking, or ruptured aneurysms (before and during surgery)
   b. Perforation and avulsion of vena cava during initial effort at aortic control
   c. Torn iliac veins during distal control of iliac arteries
   d. Ureteral transection
   e. Duodenal injury
   f. Late aortoduodenal fistula
   g. Cholesterol embolization: heart, brain, kidney, peripheral vascular system
   h. Thromboembolism

    i. Air embolism
    j. Spinal cord damage: occlusion of artery of Adamkiewicz (much more of a concern with thoracic descending aorta procedures).
2. Specific nonsurgical hazards:
    a. Myocardial ischemia and infarction (highest risk is during first 3 days after surgery)
    b. Hypovolemia
    c. Hypervolemia
    d. Renal failure
    e. Disseminated intravascular coagulation (DIC)
    f. Hypothermia

Postoperative Management Monitor transport to ICU even if patient is not intubated or receiving ventilation. Pay special attention to lower extremity pulses and perfusion, myocardial ischemia, and renal function.

Postoperative Pain Intensity Severe.

Postoperative Pain Control IV narcotics; epidural catheter with fentanyl 0.5–1.0 g/kg/h with or without bupivicaine 0.10% solution; PCA.

Postoperative Problems The most common serious postoperative complications are acute renal failure and myocardial infarction; other less common complications include bowel infarction and lower extremity ischemia. Spinal cord ischemia is rare (<1%) with infrarenal aneurysms.

Postoperative Tests CBC, coagulation profile, electrolytes, glucose, BUN, creatinine, Ca^{2+}, Mg^{2+}, LFTs, ECG, CXR, ABG.

SURGICAL PROCEDURE Ascending Aorta and Aortic Arch Surgery

1. Includes thoracic aortic surgery for aneurysms, dissection, and traumatic aortic rupture.
2. Ascending aorta surgery may also involve valvular replacement and reimplantation of coronary vessels.
3. Thoracic aortic aneurysms are classified according to location (i.e., ascending aorta, aortic arch, or descending aorta) and cause (e.g., atherosclerosis, Marfan's syndrome, infectious syphilis).
4. Don't confuse thoracic aortic aneurysms with thoracic aortic dissections (DeBakey's and Dailey's classification). In Dailey's (Stanford's) classification of aortic dissection, type A dissections involve the ascending aorta; type B dissections involve the descending aorta only. Emergency surgery recommended for type A dissection: 90–95% die in a short time without repair. Initial medical management is recommended in type B dissection.
5. Traumatic aortic ruptures due to deceleration injuries most commonly involve the descending aorta at the isthmus, but one fourth involve the ascending aorta.

Objective   Repair of aortic lesion with vascular graft to prevent aortic rupture, cardiac tamponade, aortic valve insufficiency, coronary artery compromise, peripheral vascular compromise.

Position   Supine.

Exposure   Neck to pubis.

Incision   Sternotomy.

Blood Bank Order   4–8 units PRBCs; autologous predonation and autotransfuser optional; coagulation blood products if indicated.
> *Comments:* Consider use of antifibrinolytics (e.g., aprotinin or tranexamic acid).

Estimated Blood Loss   More than 800 ml.
> *Comments:* Potential for massive blood loss.

Preoperative Studies
1. Workup based on urgency (e.g., aortic rupture may involve no workup).
2. CBC, coagulation profile, electrolytes, BUN, creatinine, glucose, ECG, CXR, echocardiography, CT scan. MRI angiography (aortic, carotid, and coronary) may obviate need for ionic contrast agents.
> *Comments:* Valvular function, coronary circulation, and ventricular function may be compromised in ascending aorta dissection and aneurysms.

Anesthetic Choices   General anesthesia. Prepare for cardiopulmonary bypass (CPB) with ascending aorta aneurysm repair and aortic arch surgery.
> *Comments:* Postoperative epidural or spinal analgesia is less advantageous for patients with sternotomy than for those with thoracotomy. Circulatory arrest may be necessary if repair involves aortic arch.

Invasive Monitoring   Left arterial line, Foley, pulmonary artery catheter (PAC); transesophageal echocardiography (TEE) optional.
> *Comments:* During repair of the ascending aorta, the right radial artery may be compromised by cross-clamping of the brachiocephalic artery. Place the arterial line on the left side. If patient's condition and time permit, place PAC before bypass is begun. If no PAC is available, surgeon should place left atrial line. TEE is useful not only for perioperative cardiac assessment but also for preoperative aortic assessment.

Aspiration Precautions   Not necessary unless an emergency procedure or patient is at risk of gastric reflux.

Queries for Surgeon
1. Requirement for or possibility of circulatory arrest?
2. Likelihood of rupture during sternotomy and thus necessity for femoral artery and femoral vein cannulation and partial CPB before sternotomy?
3. Potential for long cross-clamp time, since procedure may involve not only aneurysm repair but also aortic valve replacement and reimplantation of coronary vessels?

Estimated Surgical Time   Variable, 3 to 6 hours.

➤ **Anesthetic Considerations**
  1. Preoperative Evaluation
   Patient is often elderly, with multiple medical problems. Pay special attention to the following:
   a. Associated medical problems: peripheral vascular disease, coronary artery disease, pulmonary disease and history of smoking, renal disease, diabetes mellitus, medications, decreases in organ reserve capacity related to advanced age.
   b. Hemodynamic, cardiac, and respiratory status of patient.
   c. Laboratory workup based on urgency of procedure.
   d. In aortic dissection, pay special attention to aortic valve regurgitation, coronary insufficiency, pericardial tamponade, extrinsic airway compression, recurrent laryngeal nerve involvement, and underlying conditions such as Marfan's syndrome.
   e. In traumatic aortic lesion, pay special attention to associated injuries.
   f. In elective repair of ascending aorta aneurysm, pay special attention to proper cardiac workup (ECG, CXR, echocardiogram, dipyridamole-nuclear studies, MUGA, and catheterization).
  2. Anesthetic Goals
   a. Preoperative evaluation.
   b. Optimization of hemodynamics and protection of major organs at risk (heart, lungs, CNS and spinal cord, kidneys) if time allows.
   c. Proper setup and monitoring available: large-bore IV lines—at least two, PRBCs and other blood products, transducers, fluid warmer, autotranfuser, arterial line and PAC, IV vasopressors and vasodilators, and CPB machine and perfusionist for arch repairs.
   d. Epidural or spinal placement if it is to be used.
   e. Smooth induction to prevent hemodynamic lability lest there be an aortic rupture.
   f. As for all cases, the five major anesthetic components are paralysis, amnesia, analgesia, maintenance of autonomic control, and hypnosis.
   g. Usual laboratory monitoring on CPB: K^+, glucose, HCT, acid-base, activated clotting time (ACT).
   h. Have vasoactive drugs available for restoration of circulation after repair.
   i. Maintain intubation after surgery.
   j. Monitor transport to ICU.
  3. Anesthetic Technique
   Depends on stability of patient and disease.
   a. With ascending aorta surgery, CPB is always necessary. If patient is stable, place all monitors and lines before surgery. Use conventional narcotic cardiac induction, with cricoid pressure if indicated, while closely monitoring hemodynamics, oxygenation, and ventilation. Give special consideration to aortic insufficiency (i.e., avoid bradycardia and provide afterload reduction) in type A aortic dissection patient. Follow with conventional CPB management.
   b. Aortic arch surgery. Most often involves CPB with hypothermic circulatory arrest, although not necessarily if surgeon uses shunts to perfuse brain. Hypothermic circulatory arrest entails

(1) Deep hypothermia to 15° to 20° C.
(2) Administration of all drugs before arrest period (includes neuro-muscular blockers)
(3) Additional CNS protection (e.g., pentothal 5–10 mg/kg; steroids are controversial)
(4) Renal protection (e.g., mannitol 0.25–1.0 g/kg)
(5) Availability of coagulation factors and platelets for coagulopathy resulting from deep hypothermia.

Intraoperative Hazards
1. Cardiovascular
  a. Perioperative hemodynamic instability due to decreasing preload (hypovolemia), decreasing contractility (ischemia, congestive heart failure, tamponade), afterload changes (vasodilatation due to anesthetics), or rhythm abnormalities (bradycardia or tachycardia).
  b. Myocardial ischemia
  c. Cerebrovascular disease
  d. Aortic valve dysfunction due to ascending aorta aneurysm or dissection.
2. Blood Loss/Coagulopathy
Massive blood loss can occur during sternotomy because of aortic aneurysm, dissection, or rupture, right ventricular entry, or tear of brachiocephalic vein. Coagulopathy may result from deep hypothermia.
3. Renal
Oliguria due to inadequate perfusion, circulating blood volume, drugs (norepinephrine).
4. Respiratory
Patients often have associated pulmonary disease. Intraoperative risk of bronchospasm, inadequate oxygenation, and failure to restart mechanical ventilation after bypass.
5. Metabolic Endocrine
Monitor K^+, glucose, Ca^{2+}, acid-base balance.

Postoperative Management   ICU.

Postoperative Problems
1. Hemodynamic/Cardiac
Patients at major risk of perioperative myocardial infarction and left ventricular failure.
2. CNS Deficits
Due to embolic phenomenon (CPB, valvular procedure) and hypoperfusion (circulatory arrest and hemodynamic instability).
3. Metabolic Abnormalities
Due to diuretics, diabetes mellitus, renal dysfunction, CPB, cardioplegia, use of β-adrenergic agonists (draws K^+ intracellularly), massive transfusion. Acid-base abnormalities due to renal failure, diabetes mellitus, hypoperfusion-induced lactic acidemia, NG suctioning, diuretics, respiratory problems.
4. Coagulopathy
Most often due to or exacerbated by postoperative hypertension, hypothermia, inadequate neutralization of heparin with protamine, dilutional thrombocytopenia, functional platelet abnormality (CPB, preoperative aspirin intake), or coagulation factor deficiency.

5. Renal Failure
Due to preoperative compromise (diabetes mellitus, renovascular disease), perioperative hemodynamic instability, nephrotoxicity, hemoglobinuria contrast dyes, aminoglycosides, embolic phenomena (cholesterol, plaques).

Postoperative Pain Intensity Severe.

Postoperative Pain Control IV narcotics, epidural, or PCA.

Postoperative Tests Hemodynamic parameters, ABGs, electrolytes, calcium, BUN, creatinine, glucose, CBC, ACT, coagulation profile, CXR, ECG, urine output, and neurologic status and peripheral pulses when patient awakens.

SURGICAL PROCEDURE Thoracic Descending Aorta Surgery

Indications are thoracic aneurysms, thoracoabdominal aneurysms, and thoracic aortic dissections.

Objective Resection of diseased aorta to prevent aortic rupture.

Position Lateral decubitus or 45-degree oblique.

Incision Thoracotomy versus thoracoabdominal incision.

Blood Bank Order 4–10 units PRBCs, coagulation blood products (FFP, cryoprecipitate, platelets) if indicated, cell saver, autologous predonation. Antifibrinolytics may be considered.

Estimated Blood Loss >800 ml. May be massive.

Preoperative Studies CBC, coagulation profile, electrolytes, BUN, creatinine, glucose, CA^{2+}, ABGs, CXR, ECG, angiogram report, cardiac workup, PFTs if indicated. Cardiac workup will be based on history and physical examination and may involve cardiology consult, dipyridamole-nuclear studies, echocardiogram, MUGA scan, cardiac catheterization.

Anesthetic Choices General anesthesia, with epidural recommended in elective cases if there are no contraindications to regional anesthesia. Single-lung ventilation with double-lumen endotracheal tube (DLETT) routinely used (see Pneumonectomy [Chapter 3, General Considerations] for single-lung ventilation management).

Invasive Monitoring Foley, right radial artery line, PAC; a lower extremity arterial line is useful for monitoring distal cross-clamp perfusion pressure; if indicated, TEE, a subarachnoid lumbar catheter to maintain intracranial pressure (ICP) at <15 mm Hg and thus optimize spinal cord perfusion pressure (typically done by draining aliquots of 10 ml of CSF).
    Comments: A PAC may be misleading, especially during single-lung ventilation and if the catheter is in the left pulmonary artery. PAC not man-

datory. TEE may be useful in assessment of cardiac function, ischemia, and fluids. It is preferable to place radial artery line on right side because of proximal cross-clamp at level of left subclavian artery.

Noninvasive Monitoring   ECG leads II and V_5, temperature, twitch monitor; somatosensory evoked potentials (SSEPs).

Aspiration Precautions   Not necessary unless an emergency procedure or patient is at risk of gastric reflux.

Queries for Surgeon
1. Thoracotomy or thoracoabdominal incision?
2. CSF drainage procedure?

Estimated Surgical Time   4 hours.

➤ Anesthetic Considerations
1. **Anesthetic Goals**
   a. Preoperative optimization of cardiopulmonary status.
   b. Surgical exposure provided by adequate muscle relaxation and single-lung ventilation.
   c. Protection of organs at high risk of insult:
      (1) *Heart:* Because of high incidence of CAD in this population and because of significant demands placed on heart, tight hemodynamic control and cardiac monitoring are recommended.
      (2) *Lung:* Trauma from surgical retraction and single-lung ventilation may cause gas exchange abnormalities.
      (3) *Kidneys:* Attempt to protect kidneys with proper fluid management, mannitol, and furosemide and dopamine administration before cross-clamp is applied.
      (4) *Spinal cord:* There is a potential for ischemic injury if artery of Adamkiewicz is within aortic segment replaced.
   Comments: Protect the spinal cord by allowing slight hypothermia (34° to 35° C) during procedure, by maintaining elevated BP (e.g., systolic BP 140–180 mm Hg) during cross-clamping and the highest possible optimal distal perfusion pressure in lower extremity arterial line, by preventing hyperglycemia, restricting cross-clamping time (<20–30 min), preserving artery of Adamkiewicz, monitoring SSEPs, and by placing a temporary supraaortic to infraaortic shunt. There are conflicting data on the effectiveness of draining CSF via lumbar spinal catheter to improve spinal cord perfusion pressure.
   d. *Preparation:* Check on availability of PRBCs and other blood products. Routine anesthesia setup plus large-bore IV lines with blood administration sets and fluid warmer, vasoactive drips and resuscitation drugs, transducers for two arterial lines and PAC, autotransfuser, two epidural sets: one set for thoracic epidural and one set for lumbar CSF drainage (if done), and DLETT; bronchoscopy, SSEPs, and TEE optional.
2. **Anesthetic Techniques**
   a. *Before induction.* Routine monitors plus two large-bore IV access lines, invasive monitoring (arterial line and PAC), epidural, baseline hemodynamic values, activated clotting time (ACT), and HCT. CSF lumbar catheter optional; see *Comments* above.

b. *Induction.* Cardiac or conventional induction with attempt to keep hemodynamics stable; DLETT; confirm single-lung ventilation. N.B. avoid hypertensive or hyperdynamic response to intubation to prevent further dilatation, dissection, or rupture of thoracic aorta. Check careful lateral positioning (see Fig. 2) and recheck adequacy of single-lung ventilation.

c. *Maintenance:* relaxation, 100% oxygen on single-lung ventilation. Epidural, narcotic, and inhalation agent as indicated.

Comments: There is wide variation in choice of exact anesthetic maintenance technique.

d. *Points of special consideration:* Renal preservation with mannitol; furosemide and dopamine if indicated. Control BP before cross-clamping is done (but maintain elevated BP proximal to cross-clamp to optimize BP distally. BP distal to cross-clamp often ≤20–30 mm Hg. Monitor ICP, SSEPs, and TEE if equipment is available. Replenish circulating blood volume (N.B. significant third space losses [10–15 ml/kg/h] and potential for blood loss). Raise BP further before cross-clamping is removed. Expect decreased BP, decreased filling pressure, decreased cardiac output, acidosis, and increased ETCO$_2$ with removal of clamp. Keep intubated after surgery. Do not change DLETT to single lumen if patient's head and neck are edematous because of the potential for complete airway obstruction. Monitor on transport to ICU.

Intraoperative Hazards Most devastating complications are spinal cord ischemia (anterior spinal artery syndrome; occurs in 10–20% of cases) and acute tubular necrosis (ATN). Other complications: myocardial infarction/ischemia, bowel ischemia, bleeding, coagulopathy, aortic rupture (during induction or surgical manipulation), severe hypothermia, difficulty with single-lung ventilation, hemodynamic instability, loss of SSEPs, positioning-related problems.

Postoperative Management Monitor during transport to ICU; ensure hemodynamic stability, ventilation; epidural analgesia; neurologic examination, especially of lower extremities as soon as patient awakens; lower extremity pulses; continued drainage of CSF to maintain ICP at <20 mm Hg (controversial at best).

Postoperative Pain Intensity Severe.

Postoperative Pain Control Epidural, IV analgesia, PCA, intrapleural catheter, intercostal blocks.

Postoperative Tests CBC, electrolytes, glucose, creatinine, BUN, coagulation profile, ECG, CXR, neurologic examination, peripheral pulses.

Cardiac Procedures

SURGICAL PROCEDURE Coronary Artery Bypass Graft (CABG)

Indications CABG is aimed primarily at patients who have three-vessel disease or left main stem coronary artery disease (CAD) and CAD patients who have failed medical therapy. The only two indications for surgical management of CAD are (1) to improve prognosis in terms of cardiac mortality, that is, "quantity of life," (three-vessel disease or left main stem CAD) and (2) to improve symptoms, that is, "quality of life" (failed medical therapy).

Objective Provide revascularization to areas of the heart with restricted blood supply caused by fixed vascular obstruction.

Exposure Ankles to chin.

Incision Median sternotomy.

Preoperative Medications Morphine (0.1 mg/kg) IM; benzodiazepine, e.g., diazepam (0.05–0.20 mg/kg) PO; scopolamine (0.3–0.4 mg) PO if indicated.
Comments: Most patients tolerate such preoperative sedatives and all routine cardiac medications ordered preoperatively as well, except for aspirin. Heparin infusions often discontinued approximately 4 hours before transport to OR.

Blood Bank Order 4 units PRBCs routine; 8 units PRBCs for redo of CABG.

Estimated Blood Loss Variable. Average is 1000 ml. Depends on starting coagulation status, surgical skill, duration of procedure, effective use of cardiotomy suction, use of antifibrinolytics (e.g., aprotinin), and on whether it is a redo procedure.

Preoperative Studies CBC, PT, PTT, platelets, electrolytes, BUN, creatinine, glucose, CXR, ECG, cardiac studies. Cardiac studies might include exercise stress test, dipyridamole-nuclear studies, echocardiography, nuclear gated blood pool (MUGA) scan, and coronary catheterization.

Anesthetic Choices High-dose narcotic technique most commonly employed. Alternatives include other IV anesthetics or inhalational techniques. Typical narcotic regimen is fentanyl (50–150 µg/kg) or sufentanil (10–20 µg/kg). Benzodiazepines and scopolamine frequently are used for sedation and amnesia before and during surgery. Inhalation agents can be used for amnesia and to help control hemodynamics. Avoid N_2O, especially after cardiopulmonary bypass (CPB) because of potential for air emboli. Ketamine in small doses (e.g., 0.1–0.5 mg/kg) may help maintain hemodynamics on induction. "Breakthrough hypertension" tends to occur with pure narcotic technique, especially fentanyl. Choice of relaxant partially dependent on heart rate. Pancuronium helps to increase heart rate, and vecuronium (in combination with narcotic) helps to maintain or decrease heart rate.

Invasive Monitoring   Foley, arterial line, central venous catheter (CVC); a pulmonary artery catheter (PAC) frequently is used, or a left atrial line if indicated may be placed during surgery; TEE if indicated.

   Comments: CVC and PAC (if used) may be placed before or after induction. The following monitoring is routine: Leads II and V_5 or lead to known region of ischemia, activated clotting time (ACT), ABGs, stat blood laboratory studies (especially K^+, Ca^{2+}, glucose, HCT, platelets). Most important monitoring is visualization of heart (e.g., inotropy, arrhythmia, distension, and hypotension from cardiac manipulation can all be detected by inspection of the exposed heart). Transesophageal echocardiography (TEE) is used routinely in some institutions and never in others. Its value during CABG primarily is in assessment of regional wall motion abnormalities (RWMA), cardiac function, cardiac ischemia, volume management, and valvular function and in detection of chamber air and aortic atheroma. Postoperatively TEE is useful in diagnosis of tamponade and cardiac decompensation.

Airway Considerations   Routine.

Aspiration Precautions   Not necessary unless an emergency procedure or patient is at risk of gastric reflux.

Queries for Surgeons   Will arm veins be used for bypass grafting or will femoral vessels be cannulated? (Precludes IV cannulation in those sites.)

Estimated Surgical Time   3 to 4 hours. Time increases with number of bypass grafts performed, if there is difficulty taking patient off bypass, and in redo procedures.

➤ **Anesthetic Considerations**
   1. **Anesthetic Goals**
      a. Preoperative assessment and optimization. Focus on cardiac status:
         (1) Extent of CAD.
         Comments: Left main lesion is most severe and least forgiving.
         (2) Cardiac function or left ventricular ejection fraction (LVEF)
         (3) Arrhythmias and valvular function
         (4) End-organ involvement (e.g., CNS and renal) and associated medical problems (e.g., hypertension, diabetes mellitus, and cerebrovascular disease).
      b. Sedative premedications aimed at decreasing cardiac stress preoperatively. Order oxygen by nasal prongs with premedication and continue oxygen on transport to OR.
      c. The three most important responsibilities of the cardiac anesthetist are to ensure
         (1) *Adequate oxygen delivery* throughout procedure
         (2) *Adequate anticoagulation* while patient is on CPB
         (3) An *anesthetized state* (includes amnesia)
      d. Control airway during a smooth, controlled anesthesia induction with special attention paid to maintaining favorable ratio of myocardial oxygen supply to oxygen demand.
      e. Ensure adequate heparinization before institution of CPB.

f. Hemodilution (HCT <30%) improves rheology, especially during hypothermic CPB. Do not try to correct with blood transfusions unless HCT falls below midteens during CPB.

g. Maintain acceptable perfusion pressures (50–80 mm Hg) while patient is on CPB, especially important for brain and kidneys. While patient is on hypothermic CPB, slightly lower pressures may be acceptable in absence of cerebrovascular disease.

h. Optimize hemodynamic parameters to assist when patient is being weaned off CPB. Typically this entails transfusing back to patient the blood in CPB reservoir to increase filling pressures. Inotropic support may be required (e.g., epinephrine 5–10 μg boluses, ephedrine 5–10 mg boluses, or inotropic drips). (See Postoperative Problems below.) Use intraaortic balloon pump (IABP) early rather than late when difficulty in separating from CPB becomes apparent. Last resort for difficulty in separation from CPB is use of left ventricular assist device (LVAD).

2. Anesthetic Technique

a. Identify patient. Administer oxygen by mask or nasal prongs to patient during preparation for induction. Review recent laboratory studies. Verify availability of blood products and place routine monitors and large-bore IV access lines (two large-bore lines for redo CABGs). Titrate sedation (e.g., midazolam or small doses of narcotic) before inserting invasive monitoring.

b. Invasive monitoring. Arterial line (check BP both arms) and CVC, with or without PAC, placed before or after induction. PAC with pacing capabilities may be required in patients with sinus node dysfunction, third-degree atrioventricular (AV) block, or left bundle branch block (LBBB).

c. Have vasoactive drugs available (e.g., nitroprusside, nitroglycerin) and connected to an infusion pump if anticipating hemodynamic instability.

d. Anesthetic induction with goals stated above. Induction of very high risk or unstable patient is sometimes performed after patient is prepped and draped and surgeon, nurses, and CPB technician are available. Decompensation during induction may require emergency bypass or partial bypass.

e. Protect eyes and pressure points, since this is a prolonged procedure. Secure and ensure proper functioning of all lines after draping has been done.

f. Beware of postinduction sag in hemodynamics (due to low level stimulation) and provide good depth of anesthesia before sternotomy and mediastinal dissection. Disconnect patient from ventilator during sternotomy in the hope of preventing pneumothorax (unproven maneuver).

g. Control elevations in BP (maintain systolic at 80–120 mm Hg) before and during aortic cannulation (sternotomy and pericardial and aortic dissection are very stimulating), and then expect an impairment of venous return and drop in BP with atrial cannulation.

h. Ensure adequate heparinization (initial bolus heparin 3–4 mg/kg, ACT >400 seconds) during entire CPB period. ACT is usually done before heparinization, 3 minutes after heparin administration, every 30 minutes while patient is on CPB, and after protamine administration. ACT is kept 50% higher for patients receiving aprotinin because of "false" elevation of ACT by aprotinin. Exact limit of ACT for safe anticoagulation is unknown. However, inadequate anticoagulation while on CPB is catastrophic: clotting.

i. Turn IVs, drips, inhalation agents, and ventilator off during CPB. Continuous positive airway pressure (CPAP) (5 cm H_2O) optional. Withdraw PAC 5–10 cm to prevent pulmonary artery rupture.

j. Perform cold CPB by cooling to core temperature of 28° C and myocardial temperature of approximately 15° C during CPB.

k. Maintain mean BP on CPB in 50–80 mm Hg range. Monitor HCT, ABGs, electrolytes, ACT, and glucose while patient is on CPB.

l. While patient is on CPB, prepare drugs in anticipation of coming off CPB (vasoactive drips, protamine).

m. Before separation from CPB,
   (1) Ensure reinstitution of oxygenation and ventilation.
   (2) Ensure normalization of temperature, i.e., core 37° C and peripheral bladder temperature >35° C to prevent a significant afterdrop.
   (3) Check electrolytes and HCT.
   (4) Check functioning of monitors (i.e., transducers zeroed and leveled properly, ECG, Sao_2, Fio_2, empty Foley bag).
   (5) Ensure an acceptable cardiac rate, rhythm, and threshold for pacemaker capture. Defibrillation using 10–20 joules may be required during rewarming of patient. Antidysrhythmics may also be required (e.g., lidocaine [1 mg/kg], magnesium sulfate).
   (6) Check level of CPB reservoir. A helpful mnemonic for coming off CPB is the "5 Rs": rate, rhythm, reservoir, respirator, and reversal (for heparin).

n. After patient is successfully separated from CPB, reverse heparin with protamine (protamine:heparin ratio 1.0:1.0 of initial mg dosage. N.B. heparin 100 units = 1 mg). Beware of protamine reaction. (Major reactions are anaphylactic, anaphylactoid, or catastrophic pulmonary hypertension). Start with 1 mg of protamine and administer slowly over several minutes.

o. In the immediate post-CPB period, patients may be sensitive to supplemental narcotics, inhalation agents, and negative inotropes such as β-blockers.

p. Transport patient covered with sheets to ICU. Beware of disconnects (ETT, IVs) and runaway IVs or drips. Have oxygen (check oxygen tank pressure), ventilation bag, vasoactive drugs, monitors, and help available.

Intraoperative Hazards
1. Patient Related
   a. Hemodynamic. Patients at highest risk are those with severe left main stem coronary artery stenosis, severe concomitant valvular disease, severe ventricular dysfunction, pulmonary hypertension, or prolonged bypass time, females, and those of advanced age.
   b. Cardiac rhythm abnormalities
   c. Respiratory problems, e.g., airway management
   d. Drug reaction to protamine or to antibiotics
   e. Hematologic: bleeding diathesis after CPB

    f. Metabolic, especially K^+ and glucose
    g. Anesthetic related: intraoperative recall, PAC-related complication
2. Surgery Related
    a. Entry of right heart with sternotomy saw
    b. Rib fractures
    c. Inadequate bypass of stenosed vessels
    d. Coronary air embolism
    e. Prolonged CPB time
    f. Aortic dissection or tear with cannulation
    g. Aortic cannula inserted in carotid artery
    h. Postbypass CNS dysfunction, mostly related to macroemboli and microemboli.
3. Equipment Related
    a. Disconnection of any part of the CPB circuit
    b. Massive air embolism
    c. Reversed CPB flow
    d. Platelet dysfunction or hemolysis caused by equipment

Postoperative Management   Cardiac SICU.

Postoperative Problems
1. Hemodynamic lability
2. Cardiac abnormalities (ischemia, arrhythmias, tamponade)
3. Bleeding diathesis (medical versus surgical bleeding)
4. Respiratory (weaning difficulties)
5. Metabolic (e.g., K^+, Ca^{2+}, glucose, acid-base)
6. Pain management
7. CNS dysfunction and agitation.
    Comments: (a) Extubation is aimed at 2 to 12 hours after surgery in routine CABG. (b) Decreased BP has only two causes: decreased cardiac output (CO) or decreased systemic vascular resistance (SVR), i.e., $BP = CO \times SVR$.
    Comments: Associated medical conditions such as difficult airway (requiring intubation while maintaining spontaneous ventilation), asthma, or full stomach complicate and conflict with the cardiac-related anesthetic goals. Preoperative evaluation, optimization, and prioritization and intraoperative preparedness constitute the soundest strategy to conflicting medical conditions.

SURGICAL PROCEDURE Reexploration after Cardiac Surgery

Indications As a rule of thumb, if blood loss is >1000 ml in the first 4 hours after surgery or >200 ml/h for 3 consecutive hours despite aggressive therapy to correct coagulopathy or if the patient is unexpectedly hemodynamically unstable, reexploration is indicated to rule out a surgical cause of the bleeding, tamponade, or graft malfunction. Essentially the decision to take a patient back for reexploration is a difficult judgment call. In a patient who is bleeding excessively and who suddenly begins bleeding rapidly and becomes increasingly more hemodynamically compromised or requires higher levels of inotropic support, reexploration is indicated. Transesophageal echocardiography (TEE) may be especially helpful if time permits and assuming echographer is reliable. Cardiopulmonary bypass (CPB) rarely may be required to repair a bypass graft, but most reexplorations do not involve CPB.

Objective Correct or rule out intrathoracic bleeding due to surgery.

Position Supine, arms abducted.

Exposure Chin to toes.

Incision Reopening median sternotomy.

Blood Bank Order 10 units PRBCs, 10 units FFP, 10 units cryoprecipitate, 10 units platelets; albumin if indicated.
   Comments: Check blood product availability as soon as you realize blood loss is significant.

Preoperative Studies When blood loss is rapid, there may be no time for any preoperative studies. However, check hemodynamic parameters to ascertain degree and cause of compromise. If and when time permits, check HCT, ACT, platelet count, PT, PTT, TT, fibrinogen level, FDP, reptilase time, PTT after 1:1 dilution with plasma, and thromboelastogram; ECG, CXR, and TEE. Release of heparin from body stores after initial normalization of ACT may cause *heparin rebound.*

Anesthetic Choices General anesthesia with paralysis. Titration of narcotics or use of inhalation agents depends on hemodynamic tolerance. For patients in extremis (BP <60 and dropping), paralysis may be all that can be offered initially.

Invasive Monitoring Arterial line, central venous catheter (CVC), pulmonary artery catheter (PAC), and transesophageal echocardiography (TEE). TEE is useful here in diagnosing the underlying problem leading to reexploration, which most commonly is tamponade, cardiac dysfunction, ischemia, hypovolemia, or a valvular problem.

Airway Considerations Patient most often will be intubated already.

Aspiration Precautions Yes. If patient is extubated, apply aspiration precautions on induction (i.e., cricoid pressure).

Estimated Surgical Time   Variable; average 1 to 2 hours.

Queries for Surgeon   Necessity for or possibility of CPB (and therefore heparinization)?

➤ **Anesthetic Considerations**
1. **Preoperative Assessment**
   Time to evaluate patient may be limited. First establish ABC's; second, pay special attention to hemodynamic parameters, extent and rapidity of bleeding, functioning of sumps, coagulation profile, perioperative course, and pre-CABG cardiac and overall medical conditions.
2. **Anesthetic Concerns**
   a. Myocardial dysfunction due to a preoperative dysfunction, tamponade physiology, hypovolemia, or myocardial ischemia or infarction. Even post-CABG patients are at risk for ischemia because of small-vessel disease, incomplete repair, or graft malfunction.
   b. Coagulopathy: Surgical versus medical cause.
   c. Urgency of need for reexploration is a judgment call that depends on whether transfusions are keeping up with losses; availability of OR nurses, surgeons, or anesthesiologist; and hemodynamic stability.
   d. Avoidance of N_2O because of the risk of air emboli after CPB.
3. **Anesthetic Technique**
   a. Call for help.
   b. Once decision to reexplore is made, proceed as quickly and smoothly as possible to OR (careful not to extubate patient or lose invasive catheters). Rarely, sternotomy is performed at bedside in ICU (to relieve tamponade).
   c. In OR, place patient on ventilator and 100% oxygen; ensure bilateral breath sounds, and paralyze and connect patient to monitors. Titrate anesthetic (e.g., volatile inhalation) as tolerated. Reexplorations are often performed on patient's bed without transfer to OR table.
   d. Have available pressors, fluids, blood products, good IV access, functioning arterial line, and fluid warmers. Ensure accuracy of arterial tracing to forestall treatment of a falsely low BP.
   e. Send for appropriate intraoperative laboratory studies (e.g., HCT, ABGs, ACT).
   f. Keep patient intubated after surgery.

Intraoperative Hazards
1. Tamponade considerations:
   a. Surgeon may need to evacuate blood before induction of anesthesia if patient is in extremis.
   b. Maintain "full and fast" hemodynamic parameters (i.e., intravascularly replete and elevated HR).
   c. Hang vasopressor epinephrine drip.
2. Hemodynamic instability after reexploration may require intraaortic balloon pump (IABP).

Postoperative Management   ICU.

Postoperative Problems   Risk of continued bleeding and infection.
   Comments: (1) Continued bleeding after reexploration most likely has a

nonsurgical cause. Consider unreversed heparin, overprotaminization, a qualititive or quantitative platelet defect, or a disseminated intravascular coagulation (DIC) process. (2) Consider administration of desmopressin acetate (DDAVP) (0.3 μg/kg) and aminocaproic acid (AmICAR) (100–150 mg/kg loading dose plus infusion at one tenth the initial dose per hour) getting hematology consult, slight PEEP, and 30-degree head-up positioning.

Postoperative Pain Intensity   Severe.

Postoperative Pain Control   IV narcotics.

Postoperative Tests   Routine. Watch mediastinal and chest tubes for blood drainage and patency.

SURGICAL PROCEDURE   Aortic Valve Replacement (AVR)

Indications   AVR indicated in
1. Aortic stenosis when patient is symptomatic and has a transvalvular gradient >50 mm Hg or valve area <0.7 cm^2.
2. Aortic regurgitation when patient is symptomatic or has evidence of left ventricle dysfunction.
   Aortic stenosis: Is classified as valvular, subvalvular, or supravalvular. Most common is valvular aortic stenosis, and the most frequent cause of it is calcific degeneration of a congenitally bicuspid aortic valve. Angina is the most frequent symptom, followed by syncope and congestive heart failure (CHF). All patients are at risk of sudden death. Normal aortic valve area is 2.6–3.5 cm^2; mild stenosis area, >2.0 cm^2; moderate stenosis, 1.0–2.0 cm^2; severe stenosis, 0.8–1.0 cm^2; and critical stenosis, <0.7–0.5 cm^2.
   Aortic regurgitation: Has various causes, including endocarditis, rheumatic heart disease, trauma, and aortic dissection. Early symptoms include dyspnea, fatigue, and palpitations. Degree of aortic regurgitation is estimated qualitatively on angiographic clearance of injected dye into the aortic root (+1 to +4).

Objective   Replace diseased aortic valve and restore adequate function to prevent death (i.e., in stenotic lesions) or further cardiac deterioration (i.e., in regurgitant lesions).

Position   Supine.

Exposure   Knees to chin.

Incision   Median sternotomy.

Blood Bank Order   4 units PRBCs; 8 units PRBCs for redo procedure (i.e., previous cardiac surgery) if necessary.

Estimated Blood Loss   Variable, 500–1000 ml.

Preoperative Studies   Routine cardiac workup (see CABG) and catheterization results. Catheterization results must include ventricular function, size of ventricle and valve area, pressure gradients, and coronary patency.

Anesthetic Choices   Narcotic technique generally used. Patients with severe valvular disease may have ventricular dysfunction and may be sensitive to anesthetics.

Invasive Monitoring   Foley, arterial line, and pulmonary artery catheter (PAC) are routine; transesophageal echocardiography (TEE) if indicated. N.B. PAC may underestimate the true end-diastolic pressure of a noncompliant left ventricle. TEE is useful in assessing prosthetic valvular function.

Airway Considerations   Routine.

Aspiration Precautions   Not necessary unless emergency procedure or patient is at risk of gastric reflux.

➤ **Anesthetic Considerations**
See CABG for routine cardiac anesthesia and cardiopulmonary bypass (CPB) considerations. Anesthetic goals depend on the major valvular lesion present:
1. **Aortic Stenosis**
   Patients with severe aortic stenosis have nearly fixed cardiac output. Anesthetic goals are to maintain sinus rhythm and an adequate mean BP for coronary perfusion, to provide adequate preload, and to avoid tachydysrhythmias. Hypotension is poorly tolerated, leading to irreversible and lethal cardiac arrest. Be prepared for a "crash bypass." Preoperative or intraoperative loss of sinus rhythm or development of tachydysrhythmia should evoke consideration for immediate cardioversion or pacing (e.g., junctional rhythm). Because the myocardial hypertrophy that accompanies aortic stenosis makes myocardial preservation during CPB difficult, myocardial ischemia may result. Perioperative mortality for valve replacement in aortic stenosis is 3–10%.
2. **Aortic Insufficiency**
   Patients may have a dilated cardiomyopathy. Maintain preload, sinus rhythm, a normal-to-high-normal heart rate (90–100), and decreased afterload to improve forward cardiac output. Preoperative use of an intraaortic balloon pump (IABP) is contraindicated, but postoperatively patient may require IABP. Patients with acute aortic insufficiency may be in extremis. Patients with chronic aortic insufficiency are generally well compensated.

Postoperative Management   ICU. Patients with mechanical valves routinely require anticoagulation; generally it is started day 1 after surgery. Many surgeons keep patients with bioprosthetic valves on anticoagulants for at least several months.

Postoperative Pain Intensity   Severe.

Postoperative Pain Control   IV narcotics in the ICU with the aim of extubation on day 1 after surgery. Intramuscular injections and aspirin are avoided because of anticoagulation started day 1 for the new prosthetic valve.

Postoperative Tests ECG, CBC, coagulation profile, electrolytes, glucose, BUN, creatinine, CXR to check for ETT position, condition of lines and chest tubes, air space disease, and pulmonary edema.

SURGICAL PROCEDURE Mitral Valve Replacement (MVR)

Indications
1. Mitral stenosis before severe symptomatic impairment is generally from pulmonary hypertension and right ventricular failure.
2. Mitral regurgitation before development of significant left ventricular dysfunction.
   Mitral stenosis: Is almost always due to rheumatic heart disease. Natural course is progressive pulmonary edema, dyspnea, palpitations, and hemoptysis. Normal valve area is 4–6 cm^2. Mitral stenosis is classified as mild with valve area of 1.5–2.5 cm^2, as moderate with valve area of 1.1–1.5 cm^2, and as critical with valve area ≤1.0 cm^2.
   Mitral regurgitation: Causes include rheumatic disease, bacterial endocarditis, or papillary muscle dysfunction due to ischemia. Degree of regurgitation (semiquantitative) is determined by angiography (scale 1+ to 4+). Patients present with worsening symptoms of left- and right-sided heart failure.

Objective Replacement of diseased valve to improve functional status or to prevent further cardiac deterioration.

Position Supine.

Exposure Chin to knees.

Incision Median sternotomy.

Blood Bank Order 4 units PRBCs; 8 units PRBCs for repeat MVR if necessary.

Estimated Blood Loss 500–1000 ml.

Preoperative Studies Cardiac workup (see CABG) and catheterization results.

Anesthetic Choices Narcotic technique (e.g., fentanyl 25–150 μg/kg) is most common.
   Comments: Patients with mitral valve disease are sensitive to anesthetics because of reserve and ventricular dysfunction. Small doses of ketamine (10–50 mg) IV are sometimes useful for sustaining hemodynamics during induction. Choice of relaxant on induction depends on heart rate and need for sympathomimetic effect. Avoid use of N$_2$O because of its potential for exacerbating pulmonary hypertension.

Invasive Monitoring Foley, arterial lines, pulmonary artery catheter (PAC), transesophageal echocardiography (TEE). TEE is useful in assessing valvular and cardiac function.

Airway Consideration   Routine.

Aspiration Precautions   Not necessary unless it is an emergency procedure or the patient is at risk for gastric reflux. If aspiration precautions are necessary, consider

1. Antacids (H_2 receptor blockers) or metoclopramide or cisapride (gastrokinetic agents).
2. A modified rapid sequence of induction (cricoid pressure with a controlled, slow induction involving mask ventilation) to avoid precipitous hemodynamic changes.

► **Anesthetic Considerations**

See CABG discussion for routine cardiac anesthesia and cardiopulmonary bypass (CPB) considerations. Postoperative anticoagulation routinely is required day 1 after MVR.

1. **Mitral Regurgitation**

    Attempt to maintain sinus rhythm (although not usually possible), a decreased afterload, and a normal-to-high heart rate. Induction should proceed in a slow, controlled fashion. It may be useful to have inotrope and vasodilator drips prepared. Mitral stenosis patients are less of a challenge to wean from bypass than mitral regurgitation patients are. Major concerns in mitral regurgitation patients after bypass include left and right ventricle failure. Left ventricle failure may occur in mitral regurgitation patients after MVR because the left ventricle must generate higher pressures since it no longer ejects part of its output backwards through a low-pressure incompetent valve. Major goals of therapy are to decrease afterload with nitroprusside and to improve inotropy. Early use of the intraaortic balloon pump (IABP) is recommended. Right ventricle failure occurs because of pulmonary hypertension. Measures to alleviate replacement valve (RV) failure include adequate oxygenation, hyperventilation, rewarming, vasodilators, inotropic support such as dobutamine, and more specific pulmonary vasodilators such as prostaglandin E, prostacyclin, or nitric oxide (still investigational). Morbidity and mortality are higher with MVR than with CABG.

2. **Mitral Stenosis**

    Patients generally have a protected left ventricle: the right side of the heart is more compromised than the left is. Major goals are maintenance of normal sinus rhythm, adequate preload, and slow-to-normal heart rate (to allow left ventricle filling and measures to decrease pulmonary hypertension (e.g., avoidance of respiratory acidosis). Pulmonary capillary wedge pressure (PCWP) is not equivalent to left ventricular end diastolic pressure (LVEDP).

Estimated Surgical Time   3 to 5 hours.

Postoperative Pain Intensity   Severe.

Postoperative Pain Control   Parenteral narcotics, e.g., morphine, fentanyl. Neuroaxial techniques are rarely used because of fear of epidural hematoma. Neuroaxial technique can be used, however, when coagulation parameters have returned to normal (e.g., 24 hours after surgery). Two postoperative sedation techniques increasingly used are (1) continuous infusion of propofol combined with small narcotic doses and (2) patient-controlled anesthesia (PCA).

SURGICAL PROCEDURE Cardiac Transplantation

Indications No longer experimental. Patients are in end-stage cardiac failure. Generally they have global dilatation of all four cardiac chambers. The cause of global dilated cardiomyopathy commonly is viral, ischemic, or idiopathic. Patients fit New York Heart Association Class IV description and generally have left ventricle ejection fractions (LVEFs) between 10% and 20%.

Objective Replacement of a severely decompensated heart with a healthy, normally functioning heart.

Position Supine.

Exposure Knees to chin.

Incision Median sternotomy.

Blood Bank Order As per coronary artery bypass graft (CABG): 4 units PRBCs; 8 units PRBCs for redo operations. Consider using antifibrinolytics.

Estimated Blood Loss 1000 ml. Expect greater blood loss if there has been previous cardiac surgery.

Preoperative Laboratory Studies Cardiac workup as for CABG. Pay special attention to failing organs (e.g., liver, kidneys, lungs).

Anesthetic Choices Narcotic technique. Typically involves the use of a narcotic (e.g., fentanyl or sufentanil), a relaxant (e.g., pancuronium), and an amnestic (e.g., midazolam). N.B. The rapid administration of a benzodiazepine on top of a narcotic may cause major hemodynamic compromise in a hemodynamically tenuous cardiac patient. Keep small doses of ketamine (0.5 mg/kg or less) and a vasopressor drip available during induction to support BP if necessary.

Invasive Monitoring Foley, arterial line, central venous catheter (CVC); pulmonary artery catheter (PAC) and transesophageal echocardiography (TEE) if indicated. PAC rarely placed before bypass, but it can be useful after bypass. Thus the CVC should be an introducer sheath. PAC is passed only to the level of the superior vena cava (SVC) before bypass, and it is floated in the pulmonary artery after bypass if its use is indicated.

Airway Considerations Routine.

Aspiration Precautions Aspiration precautions are often necessary because of the emergency nature of the procedure. When aspiration precautions apply, do not do rapid-sequence induction; rather do a modified rapid sequence induction (cricoid pressure with a controlled, slow induction involving mask ventilation). Preoperative antacids (nonparticulate and an H_2-blocker), with or without a gastromimetic agent (e.g., cisapride), are indicated.

➤ Anesthetic Considerations

1. **Features Unique to Cardiac Transplantation**
   a. *Selection criteria.* Absolute contraindications: malignancy, active infection, irreversible major organ system failure (e.g., hepatic, renal, pulmonary), and severe pulmonary hypertension (greater than 8 Wood units).
   b. *Donor selection.* Contraindications in donor include prolonged hypotension, cardiac arrest, cardiac trauma, requirement for significant doses of inotropes, malignancy, or systemic infection.
   c. *ABO blood type matching* of organ donor and recipient is mandatory; antigen panel testing is done as well.
   d. *Infection risk.* All patients receive immunosuppressive drugs. Pay special attention to sterile technique (especially line insertions).

2. **Preoperative Evaluation**
   Patient often is terminally ill with multiorgan involvement. Circulation may be supported by inotropic drugs, an intraaortic balloon pump (IABP), or a left ventricular assist device to bridge patient to transplantation. Pay special attention to pulmonary dysfunction (e.g., pulmonary edema, pulmonary hypertension), hepatic congestion (elevates PT and other LFT results), and renal dysfunction. Premedication should be on the conservative side (if at all). Patients are dependent on their catecholamines and maintenance of preload.

3. **Intraoperative Management**
   a. Considerations for induction
      (1) Possibility of full stomach
      (2) A fixed small stroke volume sensitive to increased afterload
      (3) A myocardium sensitive to depressants
      (4) Dependence of patient on adequate preload and a normal-to-elevated heart rate for adequate cardiac output
         Have potent inotrope (e.g., epinephrine) available, and if patient is already on inotropy, maintain administration at same level or increase it. Coordinate time of induction with surgeon's harvesting of donor heart. Administer antibiotics and immunosuppressive agents.
   b. Bypass and postbypass period.
      (1) The denervated heart is a condition peculiar to transplantation. The transplanted heart is characterized by its unresponsiveness to indirect autonomic nervous system manipulations. Vagolytic and indirect inotropes are ineffective. Only direct-acting agents are useful. Isoproterenol is often used for 1 or several days after surgery for its inotropic and chronotropic properties and its salutory properties in pulmonary hypertension. If used, a PAC is withdrawn to the SVC level before bypass. After bypass, the circulatory parameters are different than those in effect before bypass. Two reasons for difficulty coming off bypass or difficulty during the postoperative period are
         (a) Donor organ dysfunction (due to ischemia, injury, poor myocardial preservation, underlying cardiac disease), or prolonged harvest-to-transplantation time)

  (b) Pulmonary hypertension with or without right-sided heart failure (the most common cause for cardiac decompensation)
 (2) The PAC and TEE are useful in the difficult-to-separate-from-CPB patient. Recommended approach to pulmonary hypertension:
  (a) Adequate depth of anesthesia
  (b) Hyperventilation
  (c) Good oxygenation
  (d) Avoidance of acidosis
  (e) Maintenance in sinus rhythm with a higher than normal heart rate
  (f) Pulmonary vasodilators (e.g., nitroglycerine, calcium channel blocker, prostaglandin E, or prostacyclin)
  (g) Inotropes (e.g., isoproterenol or dobutamine).
  (h) Intraaortic balloon pump (IABP)

Postoperative Management ICU in isolation unit.

Postoperative Problems Related to preoperative status (e.g., renal dysfunction, which is further aggravated by cyclosporine) and poor hepatic and coagulation status (hepatic congestion due to preoperative heart failure). Most patients do remarkably well and can be extubated day 1 after surgery.

Postoperative Pain Intensity Severe.

Postoperative Pain Control Parenteral narcotics.

SURGICAL PROCEDURE Ventricular Septal Defect (VSD) Repair

Objective Closure of septal defect to prevent further cardiopulmonary deterioration. Small VSDs tend to close spontaneously with age: surgery is generally not required. Large defects cause pulmonary hypertension. Early repair (within 1 year of diagnosis) is recommended. Hole is usually repaired with Dacron patch; surgical approach is via right atrium.

Position Supine.

Exposure Chin to knees.

Incision Median sternotomy.

Blood Bank Order 4 units PRBCs (adult); 2 units PRBCs (child).

Estimated Blood Loss Age dependent. For adults, 500–1000 ml.

Preoperative Studies CBC, coagulation profile, electrolytes, Ca^{2+}, BUN, creatinine, CXR, ECG, cardiac workup. Cardiac workup may consist of echocardiogram and cardiac catheterization.

Anesthetic Choices Pediatric cardiac anesthetic. See step 3.d under Anesthetic Considerations below.

Invasive Monitoring   Arterial line, central venous catheter (CVC), and in adults pulmonary artery catheter (PAC); transesophageal echocardiography (TEE) if indicated. TEE can be helpful in detecting interchamber shunts. In small infants, central venous access is achieved via jugular veins. If central venous access is not obtained, intraoperative fluid management may be based on observation of the heart, and the right and left atrial catheters may be placed by the surgeon at the end of cardiopulmonary bypass (CPB) for pressure and fluid management.

Airway Considerations   Routine.

Aspiration Precautions   Not necessary unless it is an emergency procedure or the patient is at risk of gastric reflux.

Queries for Surgeon   Will there be a need for circulatory arrest? Circulatory arrest may be needed to improve exposure that is hindered by intracardiac return of blood during bypass. Cooling to 16° to 18° C is required for cerebral protection during circulatory arrest. Profound hypothermia with circulatory arrest is achieved by placing ice bags around the patient's head (protect ears with ear muffs) and administering vasodilators to accelerate surface cooling, barbiturates to protect brain (use controversial at best), mannitol and furosemide to protect kidneys, and a relaxant before circulation is arrested.

Estimated Surgical Time   3 to 4 hours.

Anesthetic Considerations
1. Preoperative Assessment
  Pay special attention to child's general constitutional status (growth, weight, percentiles), pulmonary status (exercise tolerance), and cardiovascular status (presence of congestive heart failure).
2. Anesthetic Concerns
  a. VSD produces a left-to-right shunt that can result in cardiac failure. Avoid cardiac depression.
  b. If the VSD is small, flow is limited by size of defect. If the VSD is large, flow is determined by the pulmonary vascular resistance to systemic vascular resistance (PVR:SVR) ratio. With pulmonary/systemic ratio of blood flow ($\dot{Q}P/\dot{Q}S$) greater than 2, pulmonary hypertension occurs. Avoid increases in pulmonary vascular resistance.
  c. VSD is regarded as a noncyanotic congenital heart defect. Increased severity or exacerbation of pulmonary hypertension may reverse blood flow across the defect and create a right-to-left shunt (Eisenmenger complex). Eisenmenger complex may result in hypoxia and paradoxical air embolus from air introduced into the IV lines.
  d. Optimize pulmonary pressures by avoiding hypoxia, hypercapnia, and acidosis; restoring temperature; deepening anesthesia; and administering pulmonary vasodilators. May use hemodilution to improve rheology.
3. Anesthetic Technique
  a. Premedication makes induction smoother. Endocarditis antibiotic prophylaxis is recommended.
  b. Eliminate all air bubbles in IV lines.
  c. Pediatric setup.

d. Induction. Technique depends on age of child, size of defect, and cardiopulmonary status. In the child with a small defect without congestive heart failure (CHF), inhalation-based induction should be well tolerated. However, in the neonate or the patient with CHF, IV induction is recommended. Inhalation agents such as halothane may cause cardiac depression and vasodilatation.

e. Maintenance: narcotics vs inhalation agents, paralysis, amnesia. Cardiopulmonary bypass (CPB) with or without circulatory arrest.

Postoperative Management   Patient remains intubated and sedated and is monitored in ICU. Occasionally the small child with no cardiopulmonary decompensation whose VSD is repaired quickly may be extubated in the OR.

Postoperative Problems
1. Heart block due to edema or improper surgical technique around the conduction system
2. Right ventricle failure due to preexisting pulmonary hypertension and postbypass ventricular depression
3. Tricuspid regurgitation
4. Residual shunt.

Atrioventricular (AV) pacing may be required.

Postoperative Pain Intensity   Severe.

Postoperative Pain Control   Parenteral narcotics.

Postoperative Tests   Routine tests plus cardiac echocardiography and Doppler studies; cardiac catheterization and pulmonary artery pressure studies if indicated.

SURGICAL PROCEDURE   Carotid Endarterectomy

Surgical approach may include (1) routine shunting, (2) no shunting, or (3) selective shunting. Shunting refers to the positioning of a temporary intraoperative shunt from the proximal common carotid artery to beyond the cross-clamp area in the internal carotid artery. The decision to shunt in the selective shunting approach usually is based on the patient's response to carotid clamping, which is demonstrated on an EEG with general anesthetic or by a new neurologic event in the awake patient under regional anesthesia.

Objective   To remove atheromatous plaque obstructing the flow of blood in the common or internal carotid arteries in the neck.

Position   Supine, with head turned to the side opposite the lesion. An inflatable bag or a pad should be placed under the patient's shoulders to elevate the neck.

Exposure   Homolateral skin. Prepare the groin if a graft is necessary.

Incision   Oblique incision in skin crease or slanting incision along sterno-cleidomastoid muscle (more likely).

Nerves Involved   C2–4.

Blood Bank Order   Type and screen only; crossmatch not necessary.

Estimated Blood Loss   Negligible.

Preoperative Laboratory Studies   CBC, coagulation profile, electrolytes, BUN, creatinine, glucose, ECG, CXR, angiographic carotid studies.

Anesthetic Choices   General, regional, or local. A regional anesthetic, i.e., a deep and a superficial cervical plexus block, permits awake neurologic monitoring.

Invasive Monitoring   Arterial line; transesophageal echocardiography (TEE) if indicated. Arterial line is necessary to assure moment-to-moment BP control. N.B. No neck lines (e.g., central venous catheter) on surgical side. In patients having general anesthesia, TEE may be useful for monitoring of cardiac ischemia.

Airway Considerations   Routine.

Queries for Surgeon   Heparin reversal after endarterectomy.

Estimated Surgical Time   2 hours.

▶ **Anesthetic Considerations**
  1. **Anesthetic Goals**
     a. Pay special attention to neurologic and cardiovascular systems because of associated coronary artery and peripheral vascular disease.
     b. Myocardial protection: Maintain patient perioperatively on his or her usual cardiac medications; avoid intraoperative tachycardia; monitor ECG leads II and V_5 for ischemia; maintain cardiac monitoring postoperatively.
     c. CNS protection: Maintain BP at or slightly above usual preoperative level, especially during cross-clamping; monitor CNS responses in awake patient or by EEG, if available, in patient under general anesthesia.
     d. Adequate surgical exposure: An awake patient must be cooperative. The intensity with which a patient squeezes the rubber bulb on a child's horn may indicate whether the patient retains contralateral cerebral function. If patient is asleep, prevent sudden patient movement with use of relaxants.
     e. Selection of anesthetic technique (general anesthesia versus regional) is based on several factors:
        (1) Surgeon's preference.
        (2) Patient's preference.
        (3) Surgical technique (i.e., regional anesthetic technique with awake patient is best in selective shunting approach where there is no electrophysiologic monitoring; otherwise, general anesthesia is indicated). Most important factor to successful regional anesthesia is

a cooperative patient with the ability to maintain excellent intra-operative anesthetist-patient communication.

2. Anesthetic Technique
   a. Maintain stable hemodynamics; may need vasoactive IV drips (sodium nitroprusside and phenylephrine.
   b. Check BP in both arms before placement of arterial line.
   c. Use routine induction or regional block.
   d. Maintain constant depth of anesthesia when using EEG monitoring, especially at time of cross-clamping.
   e. Maintain paralysis during general anesthesia to prevent movement.
   f. Maintain normal to mildly elevated BP during clamping.
   g. Plan immediate postoperative neurologic examination and therefore immediate postoperative wakeup.

Intraoperative Hazards
1. Myocardial ischemia.
2. Neurologic complication due to
   a. Embolic phenomenon
   b. Thrombotic phenomenon (air or clot)
   c. Low perfusion with cross-clamping of internal carotid artery
   d. Altered cerebrovascular autoregulation with resultant hyperperfusion and cerebral edema.
3. BP lability (often, old and frail hypertensive patients). BP typically increases with manipulation of vessels.
4. Arrhythmia. Carotid sinus stimulation causes bradycardia. Approach to bradycardia: Stop any manipulation of carotid; atropine and local infiltration of carotid sinus if indicated.
5. Regional technique complicated by claustrophobia, patient agitation, BP lability, especially hypertension. Benzodiazepines may cause paradoxical agitation in the elderly that requires oversedation, with consequent uncooperativeness and loss of neurologic function during examination.

Postoperative Management   ICU.

Postoperative Problems   Airway compromise by hematoma; neurologic deficit due to embolus and thrombus; labile BP (patients often require vasopressors or vasodilators after surgery); cranial nerve palsy (hypoglossal, facial).

Postoperative Pain Intensity   Mild to moderate.

Postoperative Pain Control   Routine, cervical plexus block, local infiltration.

Postoperative Tests   Neurologic examination, ECG, neck examination.

SUGGESTED READINGS
Abdominal Aortic Surgery
Lunn JJ, Raimundo HS. Anesthesia for Abdominal Aortic Aneurysm. In Tarhan S (ed). Cardiovascular Anesthesia and Postoperative Care. Chicago: Yearbook Medical Publishers, 1989.

Lusby R, Lampe G, Yeager M, et al. Surgery for Abdominal Aortic Reconstruction. In Roizen M (ed). Anesthesia for Vascular Surgery. New York: Churchill Livingstone, 1990.

Roizen MF. Anesthesia for Vascular Surgery. In Barash P (ed). Clinical Anesthesia. Philadelphia: J.B. Lippincott, 1989.

Thoracic Aortic Surgery

Kwitka G, Kidney S, Nugent M. Thoracic and Abdominal Aortic Aneurysm Resections. In Kaplan JA (ed). Vascular Anesthesia. New York: Churchill Livingstone, 1991.

Kwitka G, Roseberg JW, Nugent M. Thoracic Aortic Disease. In Kaplan JA (ed). Cardiac Anesthesia. Philadelphia: W.B. Saunders, 1993.

Nugent M, Oliver WC, Jr, Roseberg JW. Anesthesia for Thoracic Aortic Surgery. In Tarhan S (ed). Cardiovascular Anesthesia and Postoperative Care. Chicago: Yearbook Medical Publishers, 1989.

Coronary Artery Bypass Graft and Reexploration for Bleeding after Cardiopulmonary Bypass

Kramer J, Thomas S. Coronary Artery Disease. In Thomas SJ (ed). Manual of Cardiac Anesthesia. New York: Churchill Livingstone, 1993.

O'Connor JP, Ramsay J, Wynands JE, Kaplan J. Anesthesia for Myocardial Revascularization. In Kaplan JA (ed). Cardiac Anesthesia. Philadelphia: W.B. Saunders, 1993.

Raimundo HS, King RM. Coronary Circulation and Anesthesia for Coronary Artery Bypass Surgery. Chicago: Yearbook Medical Publishers, 1989.

Tinker JH, Roberts SL. Management of Cardiopulmonary Bypass. Philadelphia: W.B. Saunders, 1987.

Valve Replacement

Jackson JM, Thomas S. Valvular Heart Disease. In Kaplan JA (ed). Cardiac Anesthesia. Philadelphia: W.B. Saunders, 1993.

Moore RA, Martin DE. Anesthetic Management for Treatment of Valvular Heart Disease. In Hensley FA, Martin DE (eds). The Practice of Cardiac Anesthesia. Boston: Little, Brown & Co., 1990.

Sill JC. Anesthesia for Valvular Heart Disease. In Tarhan S (ed). Cardiovascular Anesthesia and Postoperative Care. Chicago: Yearbook Medical Publishers, 1989.

Cardiac Transplantation

Blanck T, Nyhan D, Kaplan J. Cardiac Transplantation. In Kaplan JA (ed). Cardiac Anesthesia. Philadelphia: W.B. Saunders, 1993.

Camann WR, Hensley RA, Jr. Anesthetic Management for Cardiac Transplantation. In Hensley RA, Jr, Martin DE (eds). The Practice of Cardiac Anesthesia. Boston: Little, Brown & Co., 1990.

Carotid Endarterectomy

Chemtob G, Kearse LA, Jr. The Use of Electroencephalography in Carotid Endarterectomy. Int Anesthesiol Clin 28:143–147, 1990.

Clark N, Stanley T. Anesthesia for Vascular Surgery. In Miller RD (ed). Anesthesia. New York: Churchill Livingstone, 1990.

Cucchiara RF, Messick JM, Jr, Grinson NN. Anesthesia for Carotid Artery

Surgery. In Tarhan S (ed). Cardiovascular Anesthesia and Postoperative Care. Chicago: Yearbook Medical Publishers, 1989.

Messick JM, Jr. Sundt TM, Jr. Ischemic Cerebral Vascular Disease. In Cucchiara RF, Michenfelder JD (eds). Clinical Neuroanesthesia. New York: Churchill Livingstone, 1990.

CHAPTER 2

EAR, NOSE, AND THROAT (ENT) PROCEDURES

GENERAL CONSIDERATIONS

Position   Supine; head on stabilizing headholder; arms at sides.
Exposure   Head, neck, and occasionally upper chest depending on procedure.

Incision   Depends on procedure.

Preoperative Studies   Routine.

Queries for Surgeon   Endotracheal tube (ETT) type and size preferences (RAE; reinforced; aluminum wrapped)? Nasal or oral? Use of laser? Side of mouth on which ETT may be secured? Surgeon's use of nerve stimulation? Induced hypotension required? Most importantly, how limited is patient's airway (from surgeon's knowledge of fiberoptic laryngoscopy or CT scan)? Discussion of potential problems and approaches with the surgeon is essential for a smooth and safe conduct of anesthesia.

Anesthetic Choices   General.

Invasive Monitoring   If central venous access is required, choose subclavian, antecubital, or internal jugular vein on side opposite to operative site.

Airway Considerations
1. ENT patients inherently have a greater risk of a difficult mask ventilation, laryngoscopy, or passage of ETT because their underlying disease involves the airway.
2. Special endotracheal tubes such as nasal ETT, RAE tube, aluminum-wrapped ETT, reinforced tubes, tracheostomy tube, and small ETT are often required; displacement or disconnection of ETT or breathing circuit.
3. Preoperative assessment: Tumors of the upper airways, prior radiation treatment, prior surgery, and severe trismus may pose challenging airway problems requiring that the patient be awake during nasal or fiberoptic intubation and even tracheostomy.

31

4. Surgery of the oral cavity or oropharynx may be greatly facilitated by nasal intubation.
5. After intubation, throat packs are frequently used; these packs must be counted and removed before extubation.
6. Access to the airway is limited intraoperatively; extra care must be taken to secure the ETT against extubation and disconnections, particularly when the head is turned from side to side by the surgeons during the procedure.
7. It is often not possible to use oral or transnasal esophageal stethoscopes and temperature probes during head and neck procedures. Preselect alternative monitoring sites.

Aspiration Precautions   Not necessary unless an emergency procedure or patient is at risk of gastric reflux. Anticholinergics and antacids recommended for suspected or known difficult endotracheal intubation, endoscopic procedures, or oral surgery manipulation.

➤ **Anesthetic Considerations**
   1. **Preoperative Assessment**
      Routine history, physical examination, and laboratory studies. Pay special attention to airway and surgical procedure scheduled to establish proper airway management approach (see Airway Considerations).
   2. **Anesthetic Goals and Concerns**
      a. Airway as discussed above.
      b. Shared airway with surgeon.
      c. Lack of access to head.
      d. Positioning of anesthesiologist and machine relative to patient and surgeon (most often at patient's side—long breathing circuit required).
      e. Protection of eyes against corneal abrasion.
      f. Close monitoring of ventilation.
      g. Use of epinephrine or local anesthetic solution by surgeon. Arrhythmia is a potential problem with halothane.
      h. Surgical use of nerve stimulation by surgeon to assess nerve integrity, e.g., facial nerve (requires train-of-four monitoring by anesthesiologist to maintain at least one out of four twitches).
      i. Induced hypotension (especially useful in ear surgery to decrease bleeding in surgical field).
      j. Contraindications to N_2O (namely in patients with eustachian tube blockade, otitis media). Discontinue N_2O several minutes before tympanic membrane closure.
      k. Consider use of antiemetic measures (especially for procedures in which blood accumulates in stomach or for procedures of the middle ear).

Postoperative Problems   Airway edema, laryngospasm, tracheomalacia, vocal cord injury, recurrent laryngeal nerve injury, airway bleeding (see Bleeding in Tonsillectomy & Adenoidectomy discussion in Chapter 10), tracheostomy complications, accidental extubation, pneumothorax, pneumomediastinum, nausea and vertigo due to ear surgery.

SPECIAL CONSIDERATIONS

Auriculectomy Excision of ear flap (auricle) for tumor or necrosis; considerations include head positioning and use of skin graft. **Position** Supine; neck extended and turned with head resting on cushioned headrest or headholder. Occasionally shoulders elevated on thyroid bag. **Exposure** Ear, adjacent scalp, and upper neck. In extended procedures, ipsilateral neck, face, and occasionally a skin graft site may be required. **Incision** Depends on extent of procedure.

Auriculoplasty Reconstruction of ear flap may require staged procedure and harvesting of rib cartilage. **Position** Supine; neck extended and turned with head resting on cushioned headrest or headholder. Occasionally shoulders elevated on thyroid bag. **Exposure** Stage I is entire temporoparietal auricular area and ipsilateral chest wall. Stage II is stage I area plus right thigh. **Incision** Temporoparietal and curvilinear over costochondral junction of ribs 5 through 8. **Intraoperative Hazard** Potential for pneumothorax. **Postoperative Test** Order CXR after surgery to rule out pneumothorax.

External Auditory Canal Reconstruction Reconstruction of stenotic or absent external auditory canal with placement of skin grafts over exposed surfaces. **Position** Supine; head flexed and turned. **Exposure** Auricular and temporoparietal regions. **Incision** Through auditory canal or postauricular site. **Facial Stimulation** Need for complete relaxation should be verified with surgeon. **Intraoperative Hazards** Potential for vascular (jugular vein) or nerve (facial) injury.

Inner Ear Surgery Endolymphatic shunt, insertion of cochlear prosthesis, cochleosacculotomy. **Position** Supine; neck extended and head turned. **Exposure** Periauricular and temporoparietal. **Incision** Postauricular. **Anesthetic Considerations** Hypotensive techniques; discontinuation of N_2O 5 to 30 minutes before tympanic membrane closure. **Intraoperative Hazards** Risk of facial nerve injury; CSF leak.

Caldwell-Luc Procedure Transoral (gingival buccal sulcus) penetration into maxillary sinus for ablation, diagnosis sampling, or drainage. **Intraoperative Hazards** Injury to internal maxillary artery, orbit, and infraorbital or trigeminal nerves. **Postoperative Problem** Requirement for mouth breathing.

External Ethmoidectomy or Sphenoidectomy External approach to ethmoid or sphenoid sinuses for ablation of local disease or communication with nasal cavity. **Position** Supine; shoulders elevated; neck flexed; chin midline. **Exposure** Paranasal facial region to superior brow. **Incision** Paranasal. **Postoperative Problem** Nasal packing may necessitate mouth breathing.

Osteoplastic Obliteration of Frontal Sinuses Ablation of frontal sinus and obliteration with free abdominal wall fat graft. **Position** Supine; neck extended; chin midline. **Exposure** Upper eyelid and base of nose to occiput; abdomen. **Incision** Coronal, extending from crease of right helix across anterior scalp to base of left helix behind hairline; alternative incision is above brow, right to left. **Intraoperative Hazards** CSF leak; intracranial hemorrhage; injury to orbit or upper eyelids.

Parotidectomy   Excision of parotid gland for neoplastic or inflammatory disease. **Position** Shoulders elevated on thyroid bag; neck extended and chin turned to contralateral side. **Exposure** Periauricular, face and upper neck. **Incision** Preauricular area to mastoid with secondary incision from mastoid tip to midsubmandibular region. **Intraoperative Hazard** Injury to facial nerve.

Submandibular Gland Excision   **Position** Supine; shoulders elevated on thyroid bag; neck extended and chin turned to contralateral side; occiput stabilized. **Exposure** Lower face and upper neck. **Incision** Below mandible margin in upper neck for 6 to 7 cm. **Intraoperative Hazards** Bleeding from lingual artery; injury to mandibular and lingual nerves and cranial nerve XII.

Frontal Sinus Trephine   **Position** Supine; neck extended; chin midline. **Exposure** Face to above brow. **Incision** Upper eyelid inferior to medial portion of eyebrow to upper one-third of paranasal area. **Intraoperative Hazards** Bleeding from supratrochlear vessels; injury to supraorbital nerve; injury to trochlear or superior oblique muscles.

SURGICAL PROCEDURE   Laryngoscopy

May involve use of microlaryngoscopy and laser. Only difference between microlaryngoscopy and laryngoscopy is the use of the microlaryngoscope. Anesthetic considerations are similar. The most common approach for laryngoscopy and microlaryngoscopy procedures is intubation, paralysis, and controlled ventilation.

Objective   Biopsies; vocal cord procedures such as stripping; excision of nodules; Teflon injections.

Position   Laryngoscope often suspended from a stand: patient's head and mouth fixed still.

Preoperative Studies   Routine; if there is a history of cardiac or respiratory problems, a medical workup may be in order. Airway may be compromised: Preoperative airway assessment is based most importantly on history and physical examination, although x-ray examination of the soft tissues of the neck, a CT scan, and flow-loop may be useful tests preoperatively.

Preoperative Medications   Avoid sedatives in patients who have airway or respiratory compromise. An antisialagogue such as glycopyrrolate is useful in any procedure involving airway manipulation.

Anesthetic Choices   Local with or without IV sedation; general with or without intubation. Minor procedures (e.g., vocal cord procedures) may be done with local. Local block may be done with superior laryngeal, glossopharyngeal, and transtracheal nerve blocks (N.B. resulting in a loss of gag reflex and loss of airway protection). General anesthesia is preferable for protection of airway, control of ventilation, poor patient cooperation, immobility of patient (especially important in laser surgery), and surgeon's preference.

Invasive Monitoring   Unnecessary unless warranted for associated medical problem(s).

Airway Considerations   Pay special attention to extent of laryngeal obstruction and symptoms from airway compromise.

Aspiration Precautions   Standard, except that airway may be unprotected with local anesthetic technique or general anesthetic without intubation, thus exposing patient to risk of aspiration.

Queries for Surgeon   Intubation okay? If so, secure ETT to which side? Estimated duration of procedure (to tailor anesthetic)? Use of laser?

Estimated Surgical Time   5 to 60 minutes.

➤ **Anesthetic Considerations**
1. **Preoperative Evaluation**
    a. Patients often have airway problems (e.g., tumor, vocal cord abnormality, stricture) and a history of smoking or alcohol abuse.
    b. Patient must be cooperative and a good candidate for a procedure if local anesthesia is to be used. Patient immobility is essential, especially for laser surgery.
    c. *Ventilation:* Advantages of intubation are airway protection and control of ventilation, depth of anesthesia, and patient movement. Disadvantages of intubation are partial obstruction of surgical view and potential for ETT ignition (<1%). When patient is not intubated, ventilation is provided by apneic oxygenation for short periods, spontaneous breathing, or jet ventilation. Possible disadvantages of no intubation are inadequate ventilation, loss of airway control (from laryngospasm, bleeding, secretion, fumes), barotrauma with jet, and difficulty controlling depth of anesthesia.
    d. *Endotracheal tube:* Cuff of small inner diameter (ID) (5.0–6.0) cuffed tube is filled with methylene blue tinted water. Silicone, red rubber (RR), or metal tubes are preferable to polyvinyl chloride (PVC) tubes because of their greater resistance to fire and penetration. Index of flammability (most flammable requires least oxygen for ignition): PVC>Silicone>RR (i.e., PVC most flammable). N_2O burns like oxygen in trachea.
    e. *Short procedure and strong stimulus:* Tailor anesthetic accordingly. Examples of useful agents are propofol (Diprivan), thiopental, alfentanil, volatile anesthetics, succinylcholine, atracurium.
2. **Intraoperative Management**
    a. *Airway:* Assure ability to intubate before removing spontaneous ventilatory drive on induction.
    b. *"Shared airway"* concept. Because the surgeon will want to manipulate the patient's lifeline, as a rule secure the ETT firmly to the left side since the surgeon does laryngoscopy from the right side.
    c. Closely monitor ventilation (oxygenation) since there is a risk of ETT disconnection, dislodgment, obstruction, or other forms of "sabotage." SaO_2, $ETCO_2$, and precordial stethoscope monitors are useful.

Postoperative Problems   Airway edema, bleeding; loss of airway protection until gag reflex returns; hoarse voice; tooth or neck damage from laryngoscopy; negative-pressure pulmonary edema from laryngospasm.

Postoperative Pain Intensity   Minimal to mild.

Postoperative Pain Control   Parenteral narcotics.

Postoperative Tests   CXR may be useful if pulmonary complication such as aspiration or barotrauma (e.g., pneumothorax) is suspected.

SURGICAL PROCEDURE   Laser Surgery

Poses a risk not only to the patient but also to personnel. Precautions for reducing risk of laser accident are to
  1. Place sign on door.
  2. Limit power density to <10 W and duration of bursts to <10 seconds.
  3. Prohibit dry gauzes on field.
  4. Protect eyes of patient by covering them with wet gauzes and eyes of personnel with glasses.
  5. Maintain FIO_2 <40%.
  6. Use helium or air instead of N_2O. N_2O supports combustion as well as oxygen does.
  7. Use an aluminum-wrapped, small ID (5.0–6.0) ETT and follow ETT considerations in step 1.d under Anesthetic Consideration above.
Be prepared for ignition. The ETT acts like a blowtorch with oxygen blowing through it. **Fire Drill:** Turn oxygen off; immediately remove ETT; call for help; extinguish fire with water or saline; start mask ventilation and reintubate; CXR and bronchoscopy are done. Keep patient intubated with humidified gases and start steroids.

SUGGESTED READINGS
General Considerations and Specific Considerations
Donlon J, Jr. Anesthesia and Eye, Ear, Nose and Throat Surgery. In Miller RD (ed). Anesthesia. New York: Churchill Livingstone, 1990.
McGoldrick F. Anesthesia for Elective Ear, Nose and Throat Surgery. In McGoldrick K (ed). Anesthesia for Ophthalmic and Otolaryngologic Surgery. Philadelphia: W.B. Saunders, 1992.

Laryngoscopy and Laser Surgery
McGoldrick KE, Ho M. Endoscopy Procedures and Laser Surgery of the Airway. In McGoldrick K (ed). Anesthesia for Ophthalmic and Otolaryngologic Surgery. Philadelphia: W.B. Saunders, 1992.
Van Der Spek AF, Spargo PM, Norton ML. The Physics of Lasers and Implications for Their Use During Airway Surgery. Br J Anaesth 60:709, 1988.

CHAPTER 3

THORACIC
PROCEDURES

GENERAL CONSIDERATIONS

Thoracic surgery includes pneumonectomy, lobectomy, segmentectomy, and other procedures involving thoracotomy with or without single-lung ventilation. Known risk factors for thoracic surgery are (1) advanced age; (2) poor respiratory function (FEV_1 <2.0 L or predicted postoperative FEV_1 <0.8 L; MVV <50% of predicted); (3) extensive resection; and (4) the underlying associated medical problems.

Objective Pulmonary resections are done most often for tumor excision and less frequently for infections, bronchiectasis, and parenchymal abnormalities (e.g., blebs). Bronchogenic cancers, including squamous cell and large-cell lung cancer and adenocarcinoma, are the most common neoplasms resected. Most malignant neoplasms are symptomatic. Less than a third of symptomatic neoplasms are resectable, and less than a third of patients whose neoplasms are resected survive long term. Overall 5-year survival is <5%. Since median survival of patients undergoing nonsurgical therapy is only 4 months, surgery is the major curative therapy, except for small-cell lung cancer, which metastasizes early and thus rarely is resectable.

Position Lateral decubitus position (LDP) (Fig. 2). LDP is the standard for the midlateral incision; the semisupine position, for the anterolateral incision; and the semiprone position, for the posterolateral incision. The LDP requires that special attention be paid to the face, head, shoulders, arms, and legs. In the standard LDP the down hip is flexed to stabilize the patient. A pillow is placed between the legs, and the head is supported by a pillow; thus the cervical, thoracic, and lumbar spines are aligned. Arms are extended ventrally, with a pillow between them. A roll is placed just caudad to the downside axilla, but not in the axilla because that may produce a brachial plexus injury. The patient is then stabilized with retaining straps placed across the hips. Pay special attention to eyes and ears.

Exposure Clavicle to iliac crest and from anterior midline (sternum) to posterior midline (spinous processes).

Incision The incisions used most often for entry into the thorax:

1. The lateral thoracotomy incision—anterolateral, midlateral, or postero-lateral—is used for most pneumonectomy and lobectomy procedures.
2. The median sternotomy is used chiefly for anterior mediastinal lesions and cardiac operations.
3. Other incisions, which are used infrequently (e.g., thoracoabdominal), are associated with greater morbidity.

This discussion deals with the lateral thoracotomy, incisional approach.

Nerves Involved   T2 to T8.

Blood Bank Order   T&C 2–3 units PRBCs.

Estimated Blood Loss   200 to 500 ml. Blood loss is generally not important during a simple pneumonectomy or lobectomy because of the clean plane of dissection.

Preoperative Studies   CBC, coagulation profile (PT, PTT, platelets), glucose, electrolytes Ca^{2+}/PO_4, BUN, creatinine, ECG, CXR, ABGs, and PFTs; ventilation-perfusion scan and CT scan optional.

Preoperative Medications   Patient's usual medications are given preoperatively, especially bronchodilators. Some cardiologists advocate digitalization for pulmonary resections because of the high incidence of postoperative supraventricular arrhythmias, particularly in patients with a history of supraventricular tachycardias (SVTs). Sedatives, especially narcotics, are best avoided in hypoxic or hypercapnic patients.

Anesthetic Choices   General anesthesia combined with epidural.

Invasive Monitoring   Arterial line; Foley is always useful since this is a lengthy procedure; CVC optional; pulmonary artery catheter (PAC) rarely required. Monitoring is based on patient's underlying cardiorespiratory status and complexity of thoracic procedure. A healthy patient undergoing pleurodesis or a rib resection requires no invasive monitoring. For patients with major underlying cardiorespiratory disease or who are undergoing a major thoracic procedure such as pulmonary resection, invasive monitoring is recommended. An arterial line is recommended in all pulmonary resection cases since it allows close monitoring of BP and ABGs. A CVC is not a necessity for resection procedures. The benefit of having a CVC is for central venous pressure monitoring in patients in whom the goal is to maintain a low filling pressure and to provide rapid access to central circulation for administration of drugs or to convert to a PAC. The CVC should be placed before patient is positioned, preferably on the up side of the neck to allow access to and manipulation of the line intraoperatively and to reduce the likelihood of the line's kinking while the patient is in the LDP. A PAC is used rarely because (1) there are few major fluid shifts in this procedure; (2) fluid management is uncomplicated; (3) there are no important left ventricular afterload and contractility changes; (4) the catheter gets in the way of resection; and (5) there is difficulty in interpreting the PAC's occlusion pressures and cardiac output. Pulmonary occlusion pressures are difficult to interpret because of changes made in patient's position throughout the procedure. Also, balloon occlusion of a major pulmonary artery segment (e.g., right pulmonary artery) in an already surgically clamped pulmonary artery bed (e.g., left pulmonary artery) will result in falsely low cardiac output and occlusion pressures.

Aspiration Precautions Not necessary unless an emergency procedure or the patient is at risk of gastric reflux.

Queries for Surgeon Single-lung ventilation required?

Estimated Surgical Time 3 to 4 hours.

➤ **Anesthetic Considerations**

1. **Preoperative Assessment and Optimization**

   The anesthetic management begins with preoperative assessment and optimization. The preoperative evaluation of a patient undergoing seg-mentectomy or lobectomy is the same as for pneumonectomy, since a less extensive procedure may functionally (because of infection, surgical ma-nipulation) or actually (larger resection than originally planned) turn out to be a pneumonectomy. Preoperative evaluation of such patients involves a thorough history, physical examination, and review of laboratory tests. The history and physical examination must concentrate on the respiratory system, in particular on smoking, cough, dyspnea, asthma, COPD, wheezing, sputum production, exercise tolerance, hemoptysis, and weight loss. Mild hypercapnia of noncentral origin (>45 mm Hg) indicates significant loss of pulmonary reserve. On the other hand, ABGs may be normal or close to normal despite severe pulmonary disease (e.g., em-physema). Thus PFTs are done routinely: their use is not determined by the results of the ABGs. In the event of abnormal PFTs (<2.0 L FEV_1, MVV $<50\%$ predicted, or RV/TLC ratio $>50\%$), split-lung function tests ($\dot{V}/\dot{Q}$ scan) should be performed to determine resectability. The single best predictor of inability to tolerate a pneumonectomy is a split-lung function test prediction of a postpneumonectomy FEV_1 <0.8 L. In the event of a predicted FEV_1 <0.8 L, an additional test, the pulmonary artery occlusion test, can be done to determine resectability. Lung resection is contrain-dicated if occlusion of the pulmonary artery of the involved lung results in a rise of greater than 30 mm Hg in mean pulmonary artery pressure, thus predicting right ventricular failure after pneumonectomy. However, only rarely is the pulmonary artery occlusion test performed. Hence the ultimate goal of the preoperative pulmonary assessment is to prevent a patient's being chronically ventilator dependent as a result of the resection.

   Preoperative pulmonary optimization is essential, since postoperative respiratory complications are related to the degree of pulmonary dys-function. The most important preoperative optimization measures are treatment and control of bronchospasm, chest physiotherapy for pul-monary toilet, incentive spirometry and breathing exercises, and treatment of infection.

2. **Noninvasive Monitoring**

   Routine noninvasive monitoring includes $ETCO_2$, esophageal stethoscope, Sao_2, and in cardiac patients, leads II and V_5. (Watch that leads are not in way of surgical field.)

3. **Anesthetic Concerns**

   a. Ventilation-perfusion mismatch in the LDP, which gives preferential ventilation to the up lung at the expense of the down lung, is created

and accentuated by the induction of anesthesia, paralysis, and the opening of the chest.
  b. Common induction concerns are:
    (1) Elderly patients with a tenuous cardiopulmonary status. Induction should proceed in a slow and deliberate fashion, ensuring stable hemodynamics and adequate oxygenation and ventilation. Ketamine may be a useful adjunct or induction agent for maintaining BP and providing bronchodilation.
    (2) Patients with bronchospastic airway disease. Most importantly, the patient's condition needs to be optimized preoperatively, and then the major goal is induction of deep anesthesia before intubation. Useful drugs available to the anesthetist are ketamine, IV or laryngotracheal lidocaine, and inhalation agents.
    (3) Patients with major pulmonary hypertension. Factors that increase pulmonary hypertension are hypoxia, hypercapnia, light anesthesia, acidosis, and vasopressors.
  c. *Maintenance:* provided mostly by inhalation agents, with small doses of a narcotic or regional anesthetic if indicated; 100% oxygen during single-lung ventilation. Muscle relaxation facilitates thoracotomy and avoids patient movement. Benefits from inhalation agents (rapid elimination, bronchodilation, complete anesthesia) override drawbacks (theoretical concern for blunting of hypoxic pulmonary vasoconstriction).
  d. *Emergence:* To avoid damage to bronchial stump from positive pressure ventilation, extubation is routine unless patient has specific indication for remaining intubated (e.g., preoperative respiratory failure).
4. **Fluid Management**
  The risk of pulmonary edema, which has severe consequences in pulmonary resection procedures, is high. Restrict maintenance fluids to <5 ml/kg/h intraoperatively. Slight-to-moderate intravascular contraction is preferable to overhydration.
5. **Single-Lung Ventilation**
  a. *Absolute indications* are massive hemoptysis; the need to isolate the contralateral lung from spillage (e.g., operation for lung abscess); bronchopulmonary lavage for pulmonary alveolar proteinosis; and giant unilateral cyst.
  b. *Relative indications* are bronchopleural fistula and facilitation of surgical exposure during thoracic procedures (e.g., pulmonary resections, especially upper lobe lobectomies, and esophageal and aortic surgery).
  c. *Management of single-lung ventilation*
    (1) Maintain two-lung ventilation as long as possible.
    (2) Ensure proper tube position.
    (3) Administer 100% oxygen.
    (4) Monitor Sao_2 and ABGs closely.
    (5) Maintain $V_T = 10$ ml/kg and respiratory rate to achieve $Paco_2 = 40$ mm Hg.
  d. *Single-lung ventilation techniques:* Double-lumen endotracheal tube (DLETT); single-lumen tube with endobronchial placement; or bronchial blockers (e.g., Univent tubes). DLETTs are the favored means of isolating the lungs because they are relatively easy to place and allow suctioning, administration of CPAP to the nonventilated lung, and

rapid conversion back and forth from single- to two-lung ventilation. The most common DLETT used is disposable left-sided Robertshaw (avoids right upper lobe bronchus obstruction, and absence of carinal hook reduces risk of tracheal trauma). Prepare DLETT before induction and review intubation procedure with personnel assisting. Approximate size requirements: women, 35–37 French; men, 39–41 French; although size depends on size of patient and length of left main stem bronchus. The DLETT is rarely used in pediatrics. The DLETT can be malpositioned too far in; too far out; or in the wrong bronchus. Fiberoptic bronchoscope may be used selectively or routinely (on all cases) to confirm proper DLETT placement.

6. Chest Tube Considerations
Chest tube considerations in resections other than a pneumonectomy: Two chest tubes are placed and kept under seal or suction. One tube is anterior to allow escape of air. The other tube is posterior to drain fluid. With closure of the pleural cavity the lungs are fully inflated to reverse any remaining atelectasis, and the drains should be hooked up to an underwater seal to prevent lung recollapse. After pneumonectomy a single tube is placed and never put under continuous suction, as mediastinal shift with cardiovascular collapse can occur. Mediastinal shift can occur because of positive or negative intrathoracic pressure on the pneumonectomy side. Thus, tube is generally *clamped*, and air can be evacuated or introduced to allow the mediastinum to be central.

Intraoperative Hazards
1. Intraoperative hypoxia in a patient having single-lung ventilation is a common problem and an even more common examination question. Approach:
   a. Back to basics or ABCs (airway, breathing, circulation): administer 100% oxygen; ensure presence of breath sounds on ausculation; rule out accidental disconnections or extubation; ensure proper lung compliance on bag ventilation; and ensure adequate hemodynamics.
   b. Verify proper tube position.
   c. Nondependent lung CPAP (5–10 mm Hg).
   d. Dependent lung PEEP (5 mm Hg).
   e. Occasional up-lung ventilation.
   f. Two-lung ventilation.
   g. Pulmonary artery clamping in a pneumonectomy.
2. DLETT complication: Upper airway trauma; lower airway trauma (e.g., tracheobronchial tree disruption); suture of DLETT to airway; DLETT displacement.
3. Bronchospasm.
4. Perioperative arrhythmias: SVTs and ventricular ectopy are not uncommon, especially with left lung resections (N.B. halothane is most arrhythmogenic).
5. Inability to extubate at end of procedure because of extent of pulmonary resection or pulmonary edema.
6. Bleeding.

Postoperative ICU. Given the magnitude of the surgical procedure, the potential life-threatening postoperative complications, and the limited respiratory reserve in these patients, all are monitored in the ICU postoperatively.

Postoperative Problems
1. Pain.
2. Chest tube problems (pneumothorax, subcutaneous emphysema, effusion).
3. Respiratory failure.
4. Arrhythmias (SVTs especially common) and pulmonary hypertension.
5. Surgical complications (stump or anastomotic suture release, bleeding, lung torsion, and lung infarction).
6. Cardiac herniation through pericardial window (rare).

Postoperative Pain Intensity   Severe.

Postoperative Pain Control   In view of the severe pain resulting from thoracotomy, the often poor pulmonary reserve in this patient population, and the strong indication for early postoperative extubation, most patients have epidurals for optimization of postoperative analgesia. Analgesia is provided with epidural fentanyl (10 μg/ml) at 5–10 ml/h continuous infusion. Epidural analgesia may be thoracic or lumbar. PCA, interpleural catheters, intercostal nerve blocks, and parenteral narcotics may also be used.

Postoperative Tests SaO_2 monitor, CXR, ECG, ABGs.

SURGICAL PROCEDURE   Anterior Mediastinal Mass

The same anesthesia approach is applicable to procedures for superior and middle mediastinal masses. Most anterior mediastinal masses that cause airway obstruction are lymphomas. Other causes are thyroid tumors, cystic hygromas, teratomas, and thymomas.

Objective   Biopsy or excision for diagnosis. Procedure is often accompanied by mediastinoscopy.

Position   Supine or lateral thoracotomy.

Exposure
1. Sternotomy: neck to midabdomen, to both midaxillary lines.
2. Lateral thoracotomy: anterior midline to spine posteriorly and neck to abdomen.

Incision   Median sternotomy or 4th intercostal anterolateral thoracotomy.

Nerves Involved   T2 to T8.

Blood Bank Order   T&C 2–4 units PRBCs.

Estimated Blood Loss   Generally small but can be extensive.

Preoperative Studies   CBC, coagulation profile, electrolytes, BUN, creatinine, glucose, calcium, CXR, thoracic CT scan, PFTs, ABGs, echocardiogram.

Anesthetic Choices   General endotracheal; combined general endotracheal with lumbar or thoracic epidural. Local anesthetic strongly advised for biopsy if flow-volume, echocardiogram, or CT scan is positive for upper airway obstruction.

Invasive Monitoring   Arterial line.

Airway Considerations   The mass may compromise the airway, making it difficult or impossible to ventilate the patient after induction of deep anesthesia or paralysis. If you are at all concerned about airway compromise, consider awake intubation, a slow inhalation, or IV induction; that is, maintain spontaneous respirations until chest is open. Also consider bronchoscopy to inspect trachea before induction of general anesthesia.

Aspiration Precautions   Not necessary unless an emergency procedure or patient is at risk of gastric reflux.

Estimated Surgical Time   3 to 4 hours.

➤ **Anesthetic Considerations**
  1. **Preoperative Assessment**
     a. Assess for respiratory compromise (classically dyspnea in the supine position) by history, physical examination, and laboratory studies listed above. CT scan, PFTs, bronchoscopy, and flow-volume loops in upright and supine positions are helpful in evaluating whether the mass is compromising the airway. Echocardiograms, supine and upright, are helpful for evaluating vascular or cardiac involvement even if patient has no symptoms.
     b. Consider preoperative radiation or chemotherapy to shrink radio- or chemo-sensitive masses.
     c. Superior vena caval syndrome secondary to mechanical obstruction of SVC results in head, neck, and upper extremity venous dilation; engorgement and cyanosis; respiratory symptoms secondary to airway mucosal edema; increased intracranial pressure; and dilated mediastinal blood vessels susceptible to injury.
  2. **Anesthetic Technique**
     a. Consider local anesthesia with IV sedation for diagnostic procedure (i.e., lymph node or bone marrow biopsy, mediastinoscopy).
     b. For general anesthetic, maintain spontaneous ventilation until chest is open to avoid airway collapse with loss of spontaneous ventilation.
     c. In the event of intraoperative desaturation, ensure use of 100% oxygen, ventilation with presence of bilateral breath sounds, and hemodynamic stability. If ventilatory obstruction is present, consider bronchoscopy, changes in patient position, arrangement of endotracheal tube (ETT) beyond area of collapse, or passage of rigid bronchoscope past the obstruction (need standby rigid bronchoscope).
     d. In SVC syndrome, keep patient in head-up position; avoid upper extremities for IV access; have blood available.
     e. For large, symptomatic mediastinal masses, be prepared for cardiopulmonary bypass in the event of intraoperative hemodynamic deterioration and respiratory compromise unresponsive to the above measures.

Intraoperative Hazards
1. Airway distortion due to tumor and airway collapse on induction is the most feared complication.
2. Hemodynamic or respiratory compromise and bleeding can occur during mediastinoscopy.
3. Compression of pulmonary artery or heart is rare.

Postoperative Management   ICU.

Postoperative Problems
1. Respiratory and hemodynamic compromise due to pain
2. Enlargement of biopsied tumor due to bleeding or edema
3. SVC syndrome
4. Pneumomediastinum
5. Pneumothorax
6. Tracheomalacia, bronchial leak, or bronchopleural fistula following tumor excision
7. Tamponade physiology due to bleeding in mediastinum

Postoperative Pain Intensity   Severe.

Postoperative Pain Control   Parenteral narcotics; epidural, intercostal block; PCA.

Postoperative Tests   HCT, CXR, ECG.

SURGICAL PROCEDURE   Bronchoscopy

A flexible fiberoptic scope is passed with or without an ETT in place, whereas a rigid scope is passed without an ETT. Rigid bronchoscopy is indicated for foreign bodies, massive hemoptysis, endobronchial resections, vascular tumors.

Objective   Diagnostic evaluation or therapeutic approach to tracheobronchial tree.
1. Examples of *diagnostic evaluation:* Cough with hemoptysis; persistent pneumonia; anatomic evaluation; tumor or metastatic workup.
2. Examples of *therapeutic indications:* Difficult intubation, foreign bodies, atelectasis, laser surgery, endobronchial tube placement, hemoptysis, brachyradiotherapy (i.e., high-dose local radiation therapy).

Position   Supine.

Blood Bank Order   None.

Estimated Blood Loss   Nil except for conditions associated with bleeding such as vascular tumors.

Preoperative Studies   Minimal studies would include ABGs, CBC, coagulation profile, CXR. May also include PFTs, ECG, and CT scan.

Anesthetic Choices   Simple flexible bronchoscopy often is done with local anesthesia and IV sedation; an anesthesiologist may or may not be required.

Invasive Monitoring   Not necessary.

Airway Considerations   Procedure may be performed only for intubation of a difficult airway.

Aspiration Precautions   Full stomach considerations if emergency procedure, if patient is at risk of gastric reflux, or there is hemoptysis (swallowed blood).

Queries for Surgeon   Other planned procedures (pneumonectomy, mediastinoscopy)?

Estimated Surgical Time   Less than 15 minutes.

➤ **Anesthetic Considerations**
1. **Airway**
   Include supraglottic, glottic, and subglottic structures in airway assessment.
2. **Respiratory**
   Patients often have pulmonary mechanical or gas exchange abnormalities.
3. **Noninvasive Monitoring**
   ECG, BP, SaO_2.
4. **Associated Medical Problems**
   Patients invariably have significant pulmonary disease, sometimes with other major organ involvement.
5. **Anesthetic Technique**
   Depends on diagnosis, underlying medical history, surgeon's preference, and type of bronchoscopy (rigid versus flexible). Premedication with an antisialogogue is useful, but it is best administered intravenously just before procedure (e.g., glycopyrrolate 0.2 mg). Indications for general anesthesia are a pediatric case, laser surgery, patient preference, rigid bronchoscopy. Tailor anesthetics to length of procedure. With general anesthesia, control ventilation unless contraindicated. The approaches to ventilation through a rigid bronchoscope are
   a. Apneic oxygenation
   b. Spontaneous ventilation
   c. Intermittent positive pressure ventilation to prevent inhalation of fumes (eye-piece window must be closed, and laser may not be in use).
   d. Jet ventilation precludes inhalation anesthetics and requires patient paralysis to improve chest compliance.
      Whether to use paralysis during peanut retrieval in pediatric patients is controversial. Advantages of paralysis in bronchoscopy for a foreign body are control of ventilation, the need for only light anesthesia, and the relatively easy retrieval of the foreign body. The disadvantage of paralysis is the possibility that the positive pressure ventilation will push the peanut distally.

Intraoperative Hazards
1. Inadequate oxygenation or ventilation
2. Strong stimulation with consequent arrhythmias and loss of BP control
3. Trauma to teeth, neck, and airway
4. Barotrauma
5. "Autopeep" effect from bronchoscopy
6. Creation of atelectasis with prolonged suctioning
7. Patient movement may cause severe injury (e.g., with rigid bronchoscopy or laser)
8. Damage to bronchoscope from patient's biting (very expensive)
9. Laser hazards (see Laryngoscopy discussion)

Postoperative Pain Intensity   Insignificant.

Postoperative Tests   CXR; ABGs optional.

SURGICAL PROCEDURE   Esophageal Resection

Indications   Chiefly for esophageal cancer: Squamous cell in 99% of cancers arising anywhere in the esophagus except the cardia region (esophageal gastric area), where most cancers are adenocarcinoma. Alcohol and tobacco use implicated as risk factors. Overall 5-year survival is <5% and depends on metastatic stage when diagnosed. Dysphagia, inanition, aspiration, and anemia are the principal presenting problems.

Objective   Resection of tumor to allow unobstructed swallowing for remainder of patient's life. Aim is palliation. Most resections are not curative.

Position and Incision   Position determined by surgical approach:
1. Lewis resection (right thoracotomy combined with midline upper abdominal incision): patient is supine for abdominal procedure and is turned to left side for right thoracotomy.
2. Left thoracoabdominal incision: right semisupine position.
3. Transhiatal approach (supraclavicular and midline upper abdominal incision): supine.

Blood Bank Order   T&C 4 units PRBCs.

Estimated Blood Loss   500 to 1500 ml. Esophagectomies can be accompanied by major blood loss.

Preoperative Studies   CBC, coagulation profile, electrolytes, BUN, creatinine, glucose, LFTs, nutritional assessment (e.g., albumin, total protein, magnesium, phosphate, calcium), CXR, ECG; ABGs and PFTs optional.

Preoperative Medications   Nonparticulate antacids or H_2 blockers recommended.

Anesthetic Choices   General anesthesia; combined with epidural optional.

Highest degree of pain and respiratory compromise: upper abdominal and thoracic incisions. Possible major benefit from postoperative epidural analgesia. Placement of epidural before induction does not necessitate use of epidural intraoperatively, since instillation of local anesthetic may complicate fluid management. However, intraoperative epidural use may be beneficial for decreased anesthetic requirement and decreased stress response to surgery. Intraoperative epidural use may consist of just spinal opioid (lack of sympathectomy), local anesthetic, or both.

Invasive Monitoring   Arterial line and CVC; Foley is routine because procedure is lengthy, volume resuscitation is significant, and it is useful for monitoring of hourly urine output.

Airway Considerations   Single-lung ventilation facilitates surgical exposure in Lewis and in thoracoabdominal approaches.

Aspiration Precautions   Since patients often have some degree of dysphagia, odynophagia, reflux esophagitis, and esophageal obstruction, consider aspiration precautions for most patients.

Queries for Surgeon   Surgical approach, as it impacts on positioning of patient and endotracheal tube type (i.e., single-lung ventilation requirement)?

Estimated Surgical Time   4 to 6 hours.

➤ **Anesthetic Considerations**
  1. **Preoperative Assessment and Optimization**
     Patients often have a history of smoking and alcohol abuse, inanition with consequent muscle weakness, immunosuppression, poor wound healing, and multiple nutritional deficiencies. Patient also may be on perioperative total parenteral nutrition (TPN). Continue TPN intraoperatively or change to a continuous infusion (100 ml/h) of $D_{10}W$, to prevent hypoglycemia.
  2. **Fluid Requirements and Monitoring**
     Large fluid requirements: Maintenance plus replacement for third space losses (10–15 ml/kg/h) and blood replacement. Large-bore IV access.
  3. **Temperature Maintenance**
     Because of major fluid requirements, duration of procedure, and large abdominothoracic surface area exposure, use all measures to maintain temperature homeostasis including warm room, humidified and warmed gases, fluid warmer. Cover exposed parts with blankets (with or without warming) and plastic sheets. Use warmed irrigation solutions.
  4. **Positioning**
     Pay special attention to possible nerve compressions and pressure points because procedure is lengthy.
  5. **Anesthetic Technique**
     a. *Induction:* take into account aspiration precautions, patient's cardiorespiratory and intravascular status (possibility of dehydration from inanition), and single-lung ventilation considerations (see pp. 40–41).
     b. *Maintenance:* provided by narcotics or inhalation agents or both; relaxants and an epidural optional.
     c. *Emergence:* Patients often are kept intubated for a time after surgery to ensure adequate airway protection.

Intraoperative Hazards During a transhiatal blunt dissection through the mediastinum (surgeon with hand in mediastinum) watch for hypotension and arrhythmias.

Postoperative Management ICU admission, ventilation, pain control, cardiorespiratory monitoring.

Postoperative Problems
1. Aspiration and airway edema are major postoperative concerns. Patients often are kept intubated postoperatively for 12 to 24 hours.
2. Respiratory compromise can result from lung manipulation during thoracotomy.
3. Third space losses continue to require large fluid replacement titrated to hemodynamics, central venous pressure, and urine output.
4. Arrhythmias, particularly supraventricular tachycardias, are common.
5. Problems associated with underlying medical conditions such as alcohol withdrawal, cardiac morbidity, respiratory disease (COPD or chronic aspiration syndrome), and nutritional deficiencies are common.
6. Problems related to surgery are bleeding, anastomic leak, and chest tube dysfunction.

Postoperative Pain Intensity Severe.

Postoperative Pain Control Epidural analgesia or PCA recommended. Otherwise, intercostal nerve blocks or parenteral narcotics.

Postoperative Tests CBC, electrolytes, ABGs, CXR, ECG.

SURGICAL PROCEDURE Mediastinoscopy

The same anesthetic considerations apply to an anterior mediastinotomy with an incision at the 2nd or 3rd interspace (Chamberlain procedure).

Objective Evaluation of superior mediastinum before thoracotomy to diagnose or establish resectability of a lung carcinoma.

Contraindications
1. Previous mediastinoscopy is an absolute contraindication because of the inevitable scarring.
2. Superior vena cava syndrome increases the risk of vascular damage.
3. Distortion of the upper airway increases the risk of injury to the airway.

Position Supine; reverse Trendelenburg. Head up minimizes venous engorgement but increases risk of venous air embolus.

Exposure Chin to xiphoid.

Incision Incision is made at suprasternal notch, and a tunnel is created by blunt dissection along the anterolateral walls of the trachea.

Blood Bank Order   T&S.

Estimated Blood Loss   Minimal, although the occasional accidental vascular tear could result in massive bleeding.

Preoperative Studies   CBC, coagulation profile (PT, PTT, platelets), glucose, electrolytes Ca^{2+}, PO_4, BUN, creatinine, ECG, CXR, ABGs, PFTs; ventilation-perfusion scan and CT scan optional.

Anesthetic Choices   General anesthesia is the preferred technique. Advantages are good patient tolerance, control of ventilation (positive pressure ventilation), decreased risk of major complications (e.g., vascular tear or air embolus), and surgeon's preference.

Invasive Monitoring   Arterial line is usually placed after mediastinoscopy if thoracotomy is to follow immediately.

Airway Considerations   Routine, but beware of anterior mediastinal masses. An anterior mediastianal mass may cause sudden tracheal collapse during induction of anesthesia (see Anterior Mediastinal Mass).

Aspiration Precautions   Not necessary unless an emergency procedure or patient is at risk of gastric reflux.

Queries for Surgeon   Plan to proceed with thoracotomy?

Estimated Surgical Time   Less than 15 minutes.

➤ **Anesthetic Considerations**
   1. **Preoperative Assessment**
      Because most mediastinoscopies are for evaluation of a mediastinal tumor of possible pulmonary origin, pulmonary or respiratory assessment is required.
   2. **Intraoperative Management**
      Intravenous induction and paralysis with short-acting agent. Maintenance with inhalation agents or short-duration IV anesthetics (e.g., propofol, alfentanyl). Extubation at end of procedure if not followed by thoracotomy.

Intraoperative Hazards
1. Hemorrhage
2. Pneumothorax
3. Air embolus
4. Compression of vessels (compression of aorta may produce hypotension or reflex bradycardia or both)
5. Compression of trachea
6. Recurrent laryngeal nerve injury
7. Infection
8. Patient movement resulting in any of the above injuries
9. Disconnection of endotracheal tube (common since surgeon works close to ETT)

Postoperative Management   Keep head up to minimize venous engorgement.

Also see Intraoperative Hazards.

Postoperative Pain Intensity Minimal.

Postoperative Pain Control Routine parenteral narcotics.

Postoperative Tests CXR.

SUGGESTED READINGS
General Considerations
Benumof JL, Allery DP. Anesthesia for Thoracic Surgery. In Miller RD (ed). Anesthesia. New York: Churchill Livingstone, 1990.

Fisankraft JB, Cohen E, Kaplan JA. Anesthesia for Thoracic Surgery. In Barash P et al (eds). Clinical Anesthesia. Philadelphia: J.B. Lippincott, 1989.

Tisi GN. Preoperative Evaluation of Pulmonary Function: Validity, Indications and Benefits. Am Rev Resp Dis 119:292, 1979.

Anterior Mediastinal Mass
Benumof JL. Anesthesia for Special Therapeutic Procedures. In Benumof JL (ed). Anesthesia for Thoracic Surgery. Philadelphia: W.B. Saunders, 1987.

Neuman GG, Weingarten AE, et al. The Anesthetic Management of the Patient with an Anterior Mediastinal Mass. Anesthesiology 60:144–147, 1984.

Bronchoscopy
Benumof JL. Anesthesia for Special Elective Diagnostic Procedures. In Benumof JL (ed). Anesthesia for Thoracic Surgery. Philadelphia: W.B. Saunders, 1987.

McGoldrick KE, Ho M. Endoscopy Procedures and Laser Surgery of the Airway. In McGoldrick K (ed). Anesthesia for Ophthalmic and Otolaryngologic Surgery. Philadelphia: W.B. Saunders, 1992.

Esophageal Resection
Eisenkraft JB, Neustein SM. Anesthesia for Esophageal and Mediastinal Surgery. In Kaplan JA (ed). Thoracic Anesthesia. New York: Churchill Livingstone, 1991.

Mediastinoscopy
Benumof J. Anesthesia for Special Elective Diagnostic Procedures. In Benumof JL (ed). Anesthesia for Thoracic Surgery. Philadelphia: W.B. Saunders, 1987.

Ehrenwerth J, Brull S. Anesthesia for Thoracic Diagnostic Procedures. In Kaplan J (ed). Thoracic Anaesthesia. New York: Churchill Livingstone, 1991.

CHAPTER 4

GENERAL SURGERY PROCEDURES

SURGICAL PROCEDURE Central Venous Catheter (Hickman, Port-a-Cath, Broviac) Insertion

Indicated in patients on long-term total parenteral nutrition (TPN), chemotherapy, or antibiotic therapy. As long as catheter manipulation is sterile and dedicated to one purpose (e.g., TPN), the rate of catheter-related infections is low, as opposed to the rate for CVC use in the ICU.

Objective Central line tunneled subcutaneously for long-term venous access, usually into the subclavian but may be inserted in the cephalic or internal or external jugular vein.

Position Supine; do not place roll between shoulder blades: diminishes space between clavicle and first rib. Trendelenburg.

Exposure Chest, clavicles.

Incision 1 cm incision at site of initial stick; catheter tunneled to ending site.

Blood Bank Order None.

Estimated Blood Loss None.

Preoperative Studies Routine. Venogram if anatomical abnormality of subclavian vein needs to be ruled out.

Anesthetic Choices Local, sedation optional; or general anesthetic. General anesthesia indicated for
1. Anxiety or patient or physician preference.
2. Pediatric or uncooperative patient.

Invasive Monitoring None.

Airway Considerations Routine.

Aspiration Precautions Not necessary unless an emergency procedure or patient is at risk of gastric reflux.

Queries for Surgeon Site of procedure (to avoid ECG pad placement there)?

Estimated Surgical Time 30 minutes.

Anesthetic Considerations IV access may be difficult. Short procedure. Spontaneous ventilation as opposed to positive pressure ventilation with general anesthesia (during search for central vein) may reduce chance of pneumothorax. While needle is in subclavian vein, awake patient is asked to take and hold a full inspiration to prevent air embolus.

Intraoperative Hazards
1. Pneumothorax
2. Arrhythmias. New onset arrhythmias may be from central line irritation of heart.
3. Air embolus
4. Arterial or thoracic duct and brachial plexus injury
5. Agitation or intolerance
6. Vein injury (inferior vena cava [IVC], jugular, or subclavian) with resultant hemothorax or hemomediastinum

Postoperative Pain Intensity Minimal.

Postoperative Pain Control Local anesthetic infiltration at operative site; routine.

Postoperative Tests CXR to verify CVC position and to rule out pneumothorax. May be done in OR.

SURGICAL PROCEDURE Esophagoscopy, Dilatation

Cause of stenosis can be caustic ingestion, surgical anastomosis, scleroderma, cancer, radiation, acid reflux.

Objective Stretch stenotic area of esophagus.

Position Supine.

Exposure Face.

Blood Bank Order None.

Estimated Blood Loss None.

Preoperative Studies Routine. Oral intake may be compromised or patient malnourished. Severe metabolic (electrolytes, Mg^{2+}, Ca^{2+}) or hematologic (vitamin K, iron, or vitamin B_{12} deficiency) abnormalities may be present.

Preoperative Medication Antisialagogue useful (may be administered intra-operatively).

Anesthetic Choices General with oral endotracheal tube (OETT). Topical with sedation possible.

Invasive Monitoring None.

Airway Considerations Routine.

Aspiration Precautions Patients at risk for aspiration because of esophageal mobility disorder, stenosis, or obstruction.

Queries for Surgeon Bronchoscopy too?

Estimated Surgical Time Less than 30 minutes.

➤ **Anesthetic Considerations**
1. **Preoperative Assessment**
   Associated medical problems, e.g., chronic aspiration or pneumonitis re-sulting in pulmonary disease or malnutrition.
2. **Anesthetic**
   Short procedure; pain is intense but of short duration. With general an-esthesia, aspiration precautions applicable in most patients. Rapidly elim-inated anesthetics such as inhalation agents, propofol, or alfentanil are recommended.
3. **Endoscopic Protection**
   Use bite block or relaxant drugs or both to keep patient from biting en-doscope.

Intraoperative Hazards Protect patient's face and eyes. Perforation by scope or dilators possible.

Postoperative Problems Perforation of esophagus with mediastinitis. Pyriform sinuses are common sites of perforation. This is not usually a major problem because cervical leaks tend to be contained or easily repaired.

Postoperative Pain Intensity Mild. Severe pain (especially retrosternal) sug-gests perforation.

Postoperative Pain Control Oral analgesics, if any.

Postoperative Tests Suspected esophageal perforation demands immediate Gastrografin swallow studies, followed by repair of the esophagus.

SURGICAL PROCEDURE Gallbladder Surgery

Recurrent biliary colic is predecessor: not harmful, but painful. Distinguish from cholecystitis. Gallbladder surgery includes cholecystectomy, choledochoduodenostomy, choledochojejunostomy, choledochostomy, and cholecystostomy. Laparoscopic cholecystectomy is the norm.

Objective Cholecystectomy is removal of gallbladder. All procedures to ensure patent common duct or drainage of gallbladder.

Position Supine; sometimes slight elevation of right side.

Exposure Upper abdomen, lower thorax.

Incision Subcostal or midline.

Blood Bank Order T&S.

Estimated Blood Loss Less than 300 ml.

Preoperative Studies CBC, coagulation profile, electrolytes, BUN, creatinine, glucose, LFTs

Anesthetic Choices General anesthesia, epidural optional. Regional technique alone is possible but is difficult and uncomfortable even in the healthy patient.

Invasive Monitoring None.

Airway Considerations General with oral endotracheal tube (OETT).

Aspiration Precautions Possible. Obesity is associated with reflux. Cholecystitis and narcotics delay gastric emptying.

Estimated Surgical Time 1 to 2 hours.

➤ **Anesthetic Considerations**
  1. **Preoperative Assessment**
     Usual history, physical examination, and laboratory studies. Pay special attention to degree of illness (e.g., perforated gallbladder versus uncomplicated cholelithiasis) and aspiration risk.
  2. **Anesthetic Requirements**
     Right upper quadrant (RUQ) retraction: need controlled ventilation. Surgical exposure facilitated by muscle relaxation. Limiting percent of N_2O decreases bowel expansion in prolonged cases.

Intraoperative Hazards
1. Bleeding from iatrogenic event.
2. Bacteremia.
3. Spillage of bile from iatrogenic event.

4. Very ill patient (e.g., American Society of Anesthesiologists class IV due to recent myocardial infarction) is poor candidate for cholecystectomy. If surgery is absolutely indicated (e.g., ascending cholangitis in such a patient), it may be best to perform cholecystostomy under intercostal or local anesthesia or to use endoscopic sphincterotomy to avoid a major operation and general anesthesia.

Postoperative Problems
1. Pain, a major problem because of high RUQ location of incision.
2. Respiratory compromise, especially in patients with borderline respiratory function.
3. Bile leak.
4. Retained stones.
5. Infection.

Postoperative Pain Intensity   Severe.

Postoperative Pain Control   Epidural narcotics; PCA; IM or IV narcotics.

SURGICAL PROCEDURE   Gastrectomy

Indication   Most often performed for gastric bleeding acutely requiring >5 units PRBCs. Patients often are chronically or acutely ill or both.

Objective   Remove diseased stomach or bypass a block.
Billroth I: Resection of distal stomach and reconstitution by end-to-end gastroduodenostomy.
Billroth II: Resection of distal stomach and reconstitution by end-to-side gastrojejunostomy.

Position   Supine; may prefer right arm at side.

Exposure   Nipples to pubis.

Incision   Midline universally accepted; bilateral subcostal often used, however. Possible thoracoabdominal incision.

Blood Bank Order   T&C 2 units PRBCs.

Estimated Blood Loss   Usually <500 ml.

Preoperative Studies   CBC, coagulation profile, electrolytes, LFTs, Ca^{2+}, BUN, creatinine, glucose, CXR, ECG; ABGs optional. Patient may have bleeding diathesis if a history of alcohol or NSAID use.

Anesthetic Choices   General, epidural optional.

Invasive Monitoring   Foley; arterial line and CVC optional.

Aspiration Precautions Often full aspiration precautions, e.g., with upper gastrointestinal (GI) bleeding, gastric outlet obstruction, and emergency surgery.

Estimated Surgical Time 1 to 3 hours, depending on origin of bleeding.

➤ **Anesthetic Considerations**
1. **Preoperative Assessment**
   Based on history, physical examination, and laboratory studies. Consider malnutrition, weight loss due to cancer, hemodynamic instability if patient has upper GI bleed, and associated medical problems such as alcohol abuse or NSAID use.
2. **Optimization**
   Correct acute metabolic abnormalities before surgery. With upper GI bleed, optimize hypovolemia before induction.
3. **Intraoperative Management**
   Usually full stomach, especially with upper GI bleed or gastric outlet obstruction.
   a. *Induction:* Consider hypovolemia in upper GI bleed.
   b. *Maintenance* fluid requirement is large (10–15 ml/kg/h crystalloid) with GI procedure. Ensure adequate IV access. Consider temperature maintenance and monitoring.
   c. *Emergence:* Attempt extubation if no contraindications.

Intraoperative Hazards
1. Bleeding
2. Pneumothorax
3. Pneumomediastinum
4. Splenic injury
5. Hypothermia
6. Hypovolemia due to third space losses

Postoperative Management PACU; consider ICU.

Postoperative Problems
1. Pain
2. Bleeding
3. Pneumothorax
4. Third space fluid requirements
5. Cardiovascular and respiratory complications common in the elderly population
6. Anastomotic leak

Postoperative Pain Intensity Severe.

Postoperative Pain Control Epidural, PCA, and IV narcotics are routine.

Postoperative Tests HCT, coagulation profile, electrolytes, glucose, BUN, creatinine, ECG, CXR are often in order.

SURGICAL PROCEDURE   Gastrostomy

1. Indicated in patients unable to feed by mouth but able to absorb enteral nutrition.
2. Often performed as a percutaneous endoscopic gastrostomy (PEG). PEG usually less traumatic than conventional gastrostomy.
3. Contraindicated if inadequate laryngeal reflexes: reflux.

Objective   Placement of a semipermanent tube into the stomach for decompression and feeding (sometimes advanced into duodenum for attempted reflux protection). PEG usually best.

Position   Supine.

Exposure   Nipples to groin.

Incision   Midline or left paramedian.

Nerves Involved   T6 to T10. The parietal peritoneum is innervated by the spinal somatic nerves; the visceral peritoneum, however, derives its nerve supply predominantly from the sympathetic nerves innervating the viscera (some parasympathetic as well). Requires T4 block.

Blood Bank Order   None.

Estimated Blood Loss   Minimal.

Preoperative Studies   Routine.

Anesthetic Choices   General, regional, or local.

Invasive Monitoring   None.

Airway Considerations   Routine.

Aspiration Precautions   None unless an emergency procedure or patient is at risk of gastric reflux.

Estimated Surgical Time   30 minutes.

➤ **Anesthetic Considerations**
1. Selection of patients for general versus awake (local or regional) technique.
2. Associated medical problems. Patients often debilitated and sometimes malnourished as well.
3. Short procedure.

Postoperative Pain Intensity   Mild to moderate.

Postoperative Pain Control   Parenteral narcotics. Intercostal blocks.

SURGICAL PROCEDURE   Hemorrhoidectomy

Also applies to lateral internal spincterotomy and drainage of abscesses and fistulas.

   Internal hemorrhoids are vascular pads located above the dentate line and covered by mucous membrane of the anal canal. *External hemorrhoids* are dilated venules located below the dentate line and covered by squamous epithelium.

Indications   Prolapse, pain, and bleeding.

Objective   Removal of diseased tissue, leaving minimal scarring and normal functioning sphincter mechanism.

Position   Lithotomy versus jackknife.

Exposure   Perianal area; buttocks taped outward.

Incision   Perianal skin with hemorrhoidal mass dissected from external sphincter mechanism.

Nerves Involved   Sacral roots.

Blood Bank Order   None.

Estimated Blood Loss   Minimal.

Preoperative Studies   Routine.

Anesthetic Choices   General, spinal, caudal, or local. General anesthetic by mask is acceptable for lithotomy position. Endotracheal tube (ETT) required for prone jackknife position under general anesthesia. Hyperbaric spinals for lithotomy and hypobaric spinals or caudal blocks for jackknife position work well.

Invasive Monitoring   None.

Airway Considerations   Oral endotracheal tube (OETT) if patient is prone and general anesthetic is used.

Aspiration Precautions   None unless an emergency procedure or patient is at risk of gastric reflux.

Queries for Surgeon   Lithotomy or prone jackknife?

Estimated Surgical Time   Less than 1 hour.

➤ **Anesthetic Considerations**
   1. **Preoperative Evaluation**
      Routine. Selection of regional anesthetic depends on patient's preference and ability to cooperate; position; and surgeon and anesthesiologist preference.

2. Anesthetic Goals
   a. Requires analgesia in sacral roots only for regional technique.
   b. Short procedure.
   c. Safe positioning.
   d. Minimize fluids because of pain on bearing down and tendency for urinary retention after surgery.
   e. To avoid an atonic bladder, do not give >500 ml fluid IV.

Intraoperative Hazards
1. Complications related to regional or local anesthesia, bleeding, or rectal dilatation e.g., dysrhythmias and hypertension.
2. Inadvertent extubation in prone position with general anesthesia would require return to supine position to reintubate. Therefore secure ETT well with patient in prone position and with general anesthesia.
3. Bleeding may be profuse but hidden by position and drapes and thus underestimated.

Postoperative Problem   Occult bleeding loss into rectal ampulla can be in liters.

Postoperative Pain Intensity   Mild to moderate.

Postoperative Pain Control   Narcotic analgesics usually required until patient is discharged from hospital.

SURGICAL PROCEDURE Hepatectomy, Partial

Indications
1. Primary and secondary malignant tumors and benign tumors
2. Repair of traumatic lesion
3. Resection of arteriovenous malformation
4. Resection of echinococcal cyst

Objective   Resection of portions of diseased liver. Removal of as much as 80–85% of normal liver is consistent with survival. Liver has extraordinary capacity for compensatory hyperplasia; it can regain its original weight within 6 weeks. Cirrhosis is a relative contraindication to resection. The liver has two independent components: right and left. The term *extended* implies removal of additional tissue from the contralateral liver (e.g., extended left hepatectomy). Removal of 80–85% of liver is incompatible with survival if trauma was agent: no time for compensatory hyperplasia.

Position   Supine.

Exposure   Nipples to pubis.

Incision   Midline abdominal; may require thoracoabdominal incision for right lobe extirpation.

Blood Bank Order   T&C 6 units PRBCs, 6 units FFP, 6 units platelets; keep a reserve of 2–4 units PRBCs on hand at all times. Use blood salvaging techniques.

Estimated Blood Loss   500 to 1,000 ml. Major hemorrhage may result from hepatic resection or from coagulopathy caused by dilutional coagulopathy, low platelets, hypothermia, DIC, or primary fibrinolysis.

Preoperative Studies   CBC, coagulation profile, electrolytes, BUN, creatinine, glucose, ECG, CXR, and evaluation of hepatic status. Hepatic status evaluated by LFTs, including PT, ALT, AST, and alkaline phosphatase.

Anesthetic Choices   General; regional technique optional.

Invasive Monitoring   Foley, arterial line, CVC.

Airway Considerations   Routine.

Aspiration Precautions   Not necessary unless an emergency procedure or patient is at risk of gastric reflux.

Queries for Surgeon   Extent of hepatic resection? Requires close communication with surgeon concerning anticipated blood loss.

Estimated Surgical Time   3 to 4 hours.

➤ **Anesthetic Considerations**
1. **Preoperative Evaluation**
   Based on routine history, physical examination, and laboratory studies. Pay special attention to underlying condition (e.g., hepatic trauma would require workup of hemodynamic status and associated injuries).
2. **Monitoring and Setup**
   Take into account potential for major blood loss and 3rd space losses. Prepare invasive monitoring equipment, large-bore IV access, blood salvaging techniques, fluid warmer, and humidifier beforehand.
3. **Anesthesia Requirements**
   Preoperative hepatic function must be adequate before the resection (otherwise, would not tolerate the resection). After resection, however, patient's hepatic function may be marginal, and actions of drugs that undergo appreciable hepatic metabolism (e.g., diazepam) may be prolonged. Otherwise, no special anesthetic regimen is required.

Intraoperative Hazards
1. Impaired hepatic function
2. Hypothermia
3. Hemorrhage
4. Air embolism
5. Pneumothorax
6. Vena cava compression
7. Coagulopathy
8. Cardiac arrhythmia

Postoperative Management   ICU bed; analgesia; monitor for postoperative problems listed below.

Postoperative Problems

1. Bleeding: May have surgical or medical cause.
2. Hypoglycemia: Monitor serum glucose levels as patients are susceptible to hypoglycemia.
3. Hepatic protein production: Monitor serum albumin and PT as reflection of hepatic synthetic function.
4. Check PT, ALT, AST, and alkaline phosphatase.
5. Liver failure: Reflected by hepatic encephalopathy, coagulopathy, hyperbilirubinemia, ascites.
6. Infection: Especially abscesses in area of resected liver.
7. Atelectasis: Due to RUQ retraction and surgical manipulation.
8. Mortality: Approximately 20%; caused by perioperative bleeding, liver failure, and infection.

Postoperative Pain Intensity   Severe.

Postoperative Pain Control   Intercostal blocks, PCA, epidural, and IV narcotics are routine.

Postoperative Tests   CBC, coagulation profile, electrolytes, BUN, creatinine, glucose, PT, PTT, albumin, liver enzymes, ammonia, CXR, ABGs, ECG.

SURGICAL PROCEDURE Hernia Repair: Inguinal, Femoral, and Ventral

---

Groin hernias may be direct, indirect, or femoral. *Indirect hernias* descend along the inguinal canal within the spermatic cord. *Direct hernias* protrude through a defect in the transversalis fascia comprising the floor of the inguinal canal. *Femoral hernias* descend through the femoral canal beneath the inguinal ligament. *Ventral hernias* are incisional hernias.

Objective   Repair indirect (peritoneal) sac and direct (fascial) defect.

Position   Supine; slight Trendelenburg.

Exposure   Umbilicus to pubis.

Incision   Transverse or oblique lateral parapubic.

Nerves Involved   Iliohypogastric and ilioinguinal have L1 origin. Other innervation from surrounding skin (i.e., T11 to L2), from the genitofemoral nerve, and from autonomic sympathetic and parasympathetic nerves. (Beware of vagal reaction from peritoneal or spermatic cord manipulation.) Requires T10 or higher block.

Blood Bank Order   T&S.

Estimated Blood Loss   Minimal.

Preoperative Studies   Routine.

Anesthetic Choices   General, spinal, epidural, or local. May be done on out-patient basis. Local consists of an inguinal block for inguinal hernia repair. It involves blocking the ilioinguinal and iliohypogastric nerves and providing a field block around the area of incision. Because of the large volume of local anesthetic required, use less concentrated solution and a vasoconstrictor. Beware of local anesthetic toxicity (e.g., 1–1.5% lidocaine with 1:200,000 epinephrine).

Invasive Monitoring   None.

Airway Considerations   Routine.

Aspiration Precautions   None unless an emergency procedure or patient is at risk of gastric reflux.

Queries for Surgeon   Laparotomy for dead bowel (strangulated hernia)?

Estimated Surgical Time   1 hour; shorter for pediatrics cases.

➤ **Anesthetic Considerations**
  1. **Preoperative Assessment**
     Routine evaluation plus special attention in certain cases:
     a. Patients with increased abdominal pressures (coughers, those with ascites) have increased incidence of hernias. Consider underlying medical problems in this patient population.
     b. Patient with strangulated hernia may be in a toxic condition from ischemic bowel and pain.
  2. **Anesthetic Technique**
     Regional anesthesia is preferable to general anesthesia with endotracheal intubation in patients with irritable airways and provides better postoperative analgesia. General anesthesia without intubation is also acceptable in patients with irritable airways (smokers, asthmatics, and COPD patients) and is preferable in short operations and in children. Spinal anesthesia has a faster onset and provides a denser block than epidural anesthesia does. Muscle relaxation is often used but is not essential. If general anesthesia is used, coughing on emergence might break repair. Coughing can be avoided by a regional or mask anesthetic, tracheal lidocaine (translaryngeal or transtracheal), immediately before intubation. Consider extubation with patient under deep anesthesia when appropriate or with use of IV lidocaine (1 mg/kg) on emergence.

Intraoperative Hazards
  1. Bleeding. Bleeding from inferior epigastric artery in posterior hernia wall or from rectus muscle is rare.
  2. Local anesthetic overdose.
  3. Rupture of repair during "bucking" or coughing on emergence (important and common anesthetic complication).

Postoperative Pain Intensity   Mild to moderate.

Postoperative Pain Control   Routine.

SURGICAL PROCEDURE Hiatal Hernia Repair (Belsey, Nissen, Hill)

There are two types of hiatal hernia: paraesophageal and sliding. Paraesophageal symptoms from obstruction are the same as sliding esophageal symptoms from reflux. Typical "antireflux" or "wraparound" operative procedures for repair of sliding esophageal hernia are Belsey, Nissen, and Hill procedures.

Objectives
1. Replacement of length of esophagus within abdominal cavity to restore lower esophageal sphincter pressure mechanism: creation of an antireflux valve.

Position
1. *Abdominal approach:* supine, left arm out.
2. *Thoracic approach:* full left lateral.

Exposure Nipples to pubis; flank to flank.

Incision Abdominal; midline abdominal or thoracic; level of 6th or 7th rib.

Blood Bank Order T&C 2 units of PRBCs.

Estimated Blood Loss Usually less than 500 ml.

Preoperative Studies CBC, coagulation profile, electrolytes, BUN, creatinine, glucose, CXR, ECG. Evaluation of pulmonary status because of aspiration pneumonitis episodes.

Preoperative Medications Tailor sedatives to patient's needs. Preoperative visit important to alleviate anxiety. Antacids (H_2 blockers, clear antacids) and gastrokinetic agents recommended for patient with hiatal hernia or esophageal reflux or both.

Anesthetic Choices General with oral endotracheal intubation (OETT), epidural optional. Single-lung ventilation via double-lumen endotracheal tube (DLETT) useful for transthoracic procedure.

Invasive Monitoring Arterial line, Foley; CVC optional. Invasive monitoring recommended: major surgical procedure, large fluid shifts, mediastinal manipulation.

Airway Considerations Routine.

Aspiration Precautions Full aspiration precautions since all patients have reflux or obstructive esophageal symptoms.

Queries for Surgeons Thoracic or abdominal approach or both?

Estimated Surgical Time   3 to 5 hours.

➤ **Anesthetic Considerations**
  1. **Preoperative Assessment**
     Routine plus special considerations for associated conditions such as chronic aspiration syndrome with consequent poor pulmonary reserve and for nonrelated associated medical conditions such as coronary artery disease.
  2. **Setup**
     Ensure routine setup plus equipment for single-lung ventilation, large-bore IV, blood administration IV set, temperature precautions (fluid warmer, humidifier, and prewarmed room), monitoring transducers, and regional equipment (i.e., epidural set and local anesthetic or narcotic for epidural).
  3. **Intraoperative Management**
     a. *Preinduction:* Identify patient; epidural and invasive monitoring may be placed before or after induction.
     b. *Induction:* Aspiration precautions; DLETT.
     c. *Maintenance:* Prolonged procedure. Relaxation recommended for surgical exposure and prevention of patient movement; 100% oxygen for single-lung ventilation.
     d. *Emergence:* Aim for extubation.

Intraoperative Hazards
  1. Problems related to single-lung ventilation and DLETT.
  2. *Hemodynamic compromise* or *arrhythmias* due to bleeding and mediastinal manipulation
  3. Positioning injuries
  4. Hypothermia
  5. Significant respiratory compromise after surgery associated with upper abdominal incision with or without thoracic incision
  6. Surgical injury to heart, lung, trachea, spleen, stomach, and vagus nerve
  7. Chest tube–associated problems

Postoperative Management   Overnight monitoring in ICU or PACU. Provide adequate analgesia. Continue fluid replacement and cardiac, respiratory, and hemodynamic monitoring, especially in patients with associated medical conditions.

Postoperative Pain Intensity   Severe.

Postoperative Pain Control   Epidural, PCA, and interpleural are routine.

Postoperative Tests   ABGs, CXR, ECG, HCT.

SURGICAL PROCEDURE Inflammatory Bowel Disease (IBD), Abdominal Exploration

Indications Ulcerative colitis (UC) and Crohn's disease.

Objective Colectomy is curative in UC. Toxic megacolon and other severe inflammatory states may dictate Hartmann procedure (rectum closed cephalad) and stoma for discharge of intestinal contents. Surgery can be on an emergency or elective basis. If it is emergency surgery, patient's condition is critical.

1. *Emergency procedures* are for
   a. Uncontrolled hemorrhage
   b. GI obstruction
   c. Toxic megacolon
   d. Bowel perforation
   e. Fulminant colitis
2. *Elective procedures* are for
   a. Partial intestinal obstruction
   b. Failure of medical management in IBD
   c. Carcinoma

Position Supine. Possibly lithotomy.

Exposure Nipples to pubis.

Incision Midabdominal most often.

Blood Bank Order T&C 2–4 units PRBCs.

Estimated Blood Loss 300–500 ml, but much greater if severe inflammation.

Preoperative Studies CBC, coagulation profile, electrolytes, BUN, creatinine, glucose, Ca^{2+}, ECG, CXR.

Preoperative Medications Often patient is young and apprehensive. Sedative may be useful. Avoid narcotics and anticholinergics in patients at risk of megacolon. Antibiotics and steroids most often indicated.

Anesthetic Choices General anesthesia, regional optional. Possibly with epidural for combined technique or postoperative analgesia.

Invasive Monitoring Foley; CVC may help fluid management. Consider multilumen with one lumen reserved for TPN after surgery. Arterial line recommended only if patient has toxemia. In patients in a severely toxic condition, pulmonary artery catheter indicated; it may be inserted after induction.

Airway Considerations Routine.

Aspiration Precautions Full stomach.

Queries for Surgeon Position? Rectal stump removal? Postoperative total parenteral nutrition (TPN)?

Estimated Surgical Time   3 to 5 hours.

➤ **Anesthetic Considerations**
  1. **Preoperative Assessment**
     Based on history, physical examination, and laboratory studies. Patient often is acutely or chronically ill or both. Pay special attention to associated medical problems; airway (decreased incidence of ankylosing spondylitis); hemodynamics (patient may be dehydrated, hypovolemic due to GI hemorrhage, or septicemic); metabolic abnormalities (especially potassium, Mg^{2+}, Ca^{2+}, albumin).
  2. **Preoperative Optimization**
     Extent and duration of optimization based on time available if an emergency procedure (e.g., perforation is an acute emergency, whereas obstruction is less urgent). Hemodynamic resuscitation usual even in the sickest of patients before induction (may be done in OR).
  3. **Anesthetic Problems**
     a. Full stomach considerations.
     b. Fluid requirements. Because of large exposed surface area, extensive bowel manipulation, possible underlying sepsis, and dehydration, intraoperative fluid requirements are enormous (10 ml/kg/h to cover 3rd space losses, replacement of deficits, ongoing losses, and maintenance). Guided by hemodynamics and urine output.
     c. Temperature homeostasis disturbed because of anesthesia, vasodilation, exposed gut, and fluid requirements.
  4. **Anesthetic Induction, Maintenance, and Emergence**
     a. *Induction:* Patient could be in a severely toxic condition; choice of induction agent and dosage needs careful assessment. Ketamine may be a cardiovascular depressant in a patient in a toxic condition with catecholamine depletion.
     b. *Maintenance:* Avoid N_2O in GI obstruction. Limit N_2O to <50% in most cases to permit easier abdominal closure.
     c. *Emergence:* If patient is severely ill, may choose to keep intubated; otherwise plan extubation.

Intraoperative Hazards
  1. Hemodynamic instability due to bacteremia and blood loss.
  2. Previous abdominal surgery and fistula or abscess formation may make surgery difficult, bloody, and liable to bowel perforation.

Postoperative Management   May require ICU. Indications for ICU based on extent of surgical procedure, intraoperative course, and patient's medical status. Ventilation and laboratory studies required.

Postoperative Problems
  1. Infection, especially with steroids
  2. Respiratory compromise if patient is malnourished and has a large abdominal incision
  3. Multiorgan system failure
  4. Pain management

Postoperative Pain Intensity   Severe.

Postoperative Pain Control   Epidural, PCA, and IV narcotics are routine.

SURGICAL PROCEDURE Laparotomy, Exploratory

Laparotomy may be performed on an emergency or elective basis. Indications are extensive.

Objective   Explore abdominal cavity.

Position   Supine.

Exposure   Nipples to pubis, flank to flank.

Incision   Midline abdominal.

Blood Bank Order   T&C 0–2 units PRBCs.

Estimated Blood Loss   Up to 1000 ml average unless complicating problems (e.g., bleeding diathesis).

Preoperative Studies   Routine and as indicated.

Anesthetic Choices   General or combined general and regional (T4 level). In combined epidural-general technique, may consider using epidural narcotics only, epidural narcotics and local anesthetic (e.g., bupivacaine 0.1–0.5%), or local anesthetic without narcotic.

Invasive Monitoring   Patients may require invasive monitoring if severely ill.

Airway Considerations   Oral endotracheal tube (OETT); consider awake intubation. Awake intubation indicated for full stomach with difficult airway.

Aspiration Precautions   Most often full stomach. Full stomach considerations include
1. NPO status <6 hours (adults)
2. Ileus (significant narcotic administration preoperatively, GI obstruction, significant preoperative pain)
3. Hiatal hernia or GI reflux

Queries for Surgeon   The presumed diagnosis and differential diagnosis possibilities?

Estimated Surgical Time   Depends on procedure.

➤ **Anesthetic Considerations**
1. **Preoperative Evaluation and Optimization**
   Routine history, physical examination, and laboratory studies. Pay special attention to degree of illness (e.g., early appendicitis versus shock in ischemic bowel), which dictates monitoring (which and when) and an-

esthetic administration. Time taken to optimize patient judged by weighing its benefits against the risk of delaying surgery.

2. **Anesthetic Goals and Problems**
   a. Patient population with diverse presentations.
   b. Variable duration of procedure. Can be short.
   c. Smooth hemodynamics require a versatile anesthetic approach dictated by the patient's severity of illness and associated medical problems.
   d. Muscle relaxation preferable for surgical exposure.
   e. For all significant abdominal cases, give special consideration to fluid requirements, temperature homeostasis, twitch monitoring, possible requirement for vasopressors, extubation, postoperative pain management, and possible ICU admission.

Postoperative Management PACU; may require ICU.

Postoperative Pain Intensity Moderate to severe.

Postoperative Pain Control PCA, epidural, parenteral narcotics.

Postoperative Tests Dictated by operation.

SURGICAL PROCEDURE Liver Transplantation, Orthotopic

Surgical procedure includes total hepatectomy. Anastomoses to the donor liver include suprahepatic and infrahepatic inferior vena cava (IVC), hepatic artery, portal vein, and biliary duct.
Surgery is divided into three stages:
1. *Preunhepatic.* Liver is freed-up to its vascular pedicle.
2. *Anhepatic.* IVC clamping and removal of diseased liver.
3. *Reperfusion or postanhepatic.* Anastomosis of transplanted liver.

Objective Exchange of diseased liver for healthy liver.

Position Both arms abducted.

Exposure Sternal notch to pubis.

Incision Bilateral: subcostal with cephalad extension to xiphoid.

Blood Bank Order T&C 10 units PRBCs, 10 units FFP, 10 units platelets; keep a reserve of 6 units PRBCs on hand; autotransfuser; rapid infusion device.

Estimated Blood Loss 6 to 60 units or more.
1. In adults a veno-veno bypass shunt sometimes is used to allow return of portal and infrahepatic venous circulation. This shunt decreases mesenteric congestion, improves renal blood flow, improves hemodynamics, and decreases blood loss.
2. Antifibrinolytics are used to decrease blood loss.

Preoperative Studies CBC, platelets, PT, PTT, electrolytes, BUN, creatinine,

Ca^{2+}, PO_4, Mg^{2+}, albumin, ammonia levels, CXR, ECG, viral serology, liver biopsy.

Preoperative Medications   Avoid IM injections. Hematomas form.

Anesthetic Choices   General anesthetic; avoid use of N_2O; usually high-dose narcotic or inhalation technique or both. Epidural contraindicated because of coagulopathy associated with end-stage liver disease.

Invasive Monitoring   Foley, arterial line, CVC, and pulmonary artery catheter (PAC) are standard; TEE may be used. Two arterial lines are placed: One is used for monitoring and the other for blood samples. Chemical and hematologic values or assayed hourly.

Airway Considerations   Oral endotracheal tube (OETT) and routine.

Aspiration Precautions   Full precautions because of ascites even with NPO status.

Estimated Surgical Time   Average is 8 hours.

➤ **Anesthetic Considerations**
1. **Patient-related Considerations**
    a. Underlying cause for end-stage liver failure. Associated medical problems include altered pharmacodynamics and pharmacokinetics; major fluid shifts; coagulopathy related to factor deficiency, platelet sequestration in portal hypertension, platelet dysfunction, and primary fibrinolysis; metabolic abnormalities (e.g., liver failure associated with hyponatremia; rapid correction of hyponatremia can produce central pontine myelinolysis). See also Anesthetic Considerations for Portasystemic Shunt.
    b. Administration of immunosuppressive therapy. Because risk of infection is high, pay special attention to aseptic techique.
2. **Procedure-related Considerations**
    Overall approach is somewhat similar to any major abdominal operation or a trauma requiring massive resuscitation. Major problems include
    a. Volume resuscitation
    b. Consequent risk of hypothermia
    c. Coagulation abnormalities due to massive resuscitation and lack of liver function
    d. Metabolic abnormalities: beware of sodium corrections, K^+ shifts, hypocalcemia, glucose disturbances, and metabolic acidosis
    e. Preservation of renal function. Continuous infusion of renal dose dopamine and mannitol (approximately 1 g/kg) recommended. Immunosuppression protocol followed
3. **Setup**
    In addition to the routine OR setup, have the following equipment available: warming blanket, fluid warmers on all large-bore IVs, humidifier, room warmed before induction, esophageal temperature probe and stethoscope, nasogastric tube, Foley, extra padding, PAC and arterial lines, PEEP valve, rapid infusion pump, autotransfuser.
4. **Intraoperative Management**
    a. Place IVs in upper extremity: IVC clamping.

   b. *Induction:* rapid or modified rapid sequence.
   c. *Maintenance:* isoflurane or narcotic technique. Relaxation provided with pancuronium.
      (1) *Preanhepatic.* Elevate intravascular volume to maintain cardiac output in anticipation of IVC clamping.
      (2) *Anhepatic.* Major problems:
         (a) Profound hypotension
         (b) Severe metabolic acidosis
         (c) Citrate intoxication resulting in hypocalcemia
         (d) Hyperglycemia due to blood product administration
         (e) Bleeding diathesis due to IVC clamping, mesenteric congestion, underlying coagulopathy, and massive transfusion. Veno-veno bypass helpful in mitigating hemodynamic instability, bleeding, and renal insult with IVC clamping.
      (3) *Postanhepatic.* Recirculation phase with anastomosis of transplanted liver. Major problems:
         (a) Hemodynamic instability due to acidosis, hepatic and gut metabolites, and myocardial depression. Give volume, pressors, bicarbonate, and calcium.
         (b) Hyperkalemia. Administer calcium, bicarbonate, insulin, glucose, and furosemide to treat severe hyperkalemia.
         (c) Persistent coagulopathy due to inability of "stunned" liver to be fully active.

Intraoperative Hazards
1. Massive hemorrhage
2. Hypovolemia from extensive third space losses
3. Hypothermia
4. Acidosis
5. Hyperkalemia
6. Hypoxemia. Hypoxemia may be due to atelectasis, intrapulmonary AV shunting, and acute pulmonary edema. Treat by increasing FIO_2 and PEEP.
7. Air embolism
8. Hypocalcemia
9. Renal failure. Intraoperative renal shutdown is major problem because of continuous need for blood products (for coagulopathy therapy) and consequent rising filling pressures and pulmonary edema. Best managed by intraoperative continuous arteriovenous hemofiltration (CAVH).
10. Reperfusion period may be stormy with respect to hemodynamic abnormalities and metabolic abnormalities.

Postoperative Management ICU. Full ventilatory support day 1 after surgery; patient often extubated 8 to 24 hours after surgery. Monitor hemodynamics, renal function, metabolic status, and liver function (bile output, PT, liver enzymes) closely.

Postoperative Problems
1. Bleeding
2. Metabolic abnormalities involving electrolytes and glucose
3. Renal and pulmonary abnormalities
4. Encephalopathy
5. Side effects from immunosuppressive therapy.

Perioperative acute mortality related to bleeding, surgical complication (vascular or biliary leak or obstruction), CNS edema, and herniation with severe liver failure. Subacute or longer term mortality rate related to rejection and infection.

Postoperative Pain Intensity   Moderate to severe. Liver transplant patients require less analgesia than expected, probably because of increased sensitivity to analgesic agents.

Postoperative Pain Control   IV narcotics in ICU setting.

Postoperative Tests   CBC, PT, PTT, ABGs, LFTs, electrolytes, Ca^{2+}, glucose, thromboelastogram, CXR, ECG, HIDA scan.

SURGICAL PROCEDURE   Lower Gastrointestinal Tract Surgery

Includes abdominoperineal resection, total proctocolectomy, resection of lower anterior rectum, end ileostomy, and rectopexy.

Objective   Anteroposterior resection: removal of rectosigmoid and areas of local lymphatic drainage, total proctocolectomy, lower anterior rectum resection, end ileostomy, rectopexy.

Position   Supine: lithotomy position; Trendelenburg. Because procedure is prolonged, take care to avoid pressure points. Possible injuries are ulnar and brachial plexus injury from olecranon pressure or hyperextension of arm; and peroneal nerve palsy from improper positioning, OR personnel's leaning on leg, or patient movement causing malposition.

Incision   Depends on procedure. Lower abdominal and anal approach.

Blood Bank Order   T&C 2–4 units PRBCs; keep 2 units in reserve. Autologous donation and hemodilution may be useful.

Estimated Blood Loss   2 to several units. Major bleeding may occur during perineal resection, much of it dripping onto floor. Torrential bleeding with laceration or avulsion of presacral veins.

Preoperative Studies   CBC, coagulation profile, electrolytes, BUN, creatinine, LFTs, ECG, and CXR optional.

Preoperative Medication   Preoperative visit is most important. Consider continuing patient's usual medications, with antibiotics and steroids in IBD patients as needed. Narcotic or sedative premedication is based on patient's status, but is not routinely necessary.

Anesthetic Choices   General or combined general and regional (T6).

Invasive Monitoring   Foley, arterial line, and CVC useful. Little urine in collection bag may be due to pooling of urine in renal pelvis or in bladder or to hypoperfusion from hypovolemia.

Airway Considerations Oral endotracheal tube (OETT).

Aspiration Precautions Aspiration precautions apply for patients with GI obstruction or who are at risk of gastric reflux and for emergency procedures.

➤ **Anesthetic Considerations**
1. **Preoperative Assessment**
   Routine assessment plus special attention to elderly, oncology, or inflammatory bowel disease (IBD) patients. Associated conditions and debilitation may be significant.
2. **Monitoring and setup**
   Third space losses extensive. Take all precautionary measures to avoid hypothermia: Prewarm room to 24° to 26° C; use fluid warmer and humidifier; keep patient covered; warm irrigation fluids; monitor temperature. Have transducers and adequate IV access set up before induction.
3. **Intraoperative Management**
   Identify patient. Large-bore IV access, although necessary, may be placed after induction. Is full stomach a consideration? Avoid N_2O if there is GI obstruction or if bowel distension is a consideration. Relaxation generally provided for optimal surgical exposure and to avoid deep anesthesia. Significant fluid requirements because of the third space losses (approximately 10 ml/kg/h). Combined technique useful to block surgical stimulation, reduce surgical stress, and lighten general anesthesia. Use of a local anesthetic in the epidural would increase fluid requirement, as opposed to an epidural narcotic.
4. **Miscellaneous**
   Antibiotic requirement. Keep checking blood loss and availability of blood. Prolonged procedures in Trendelenburg position with significant third space losses are associated with considerable head and neck edema. Extubation may not be indicated immediately after surgery.

Postoperative Management PACU or ICU. Decision to admit to ICU is based on extent of procedure, patient's underlying medical status, and intraoperative course. Sitting or semisitting position recommended to improve respiratory mechanism and decrease head and neck soft tissue edema.

Postoperative Problems
1. Bleeding
2. Hypovolemia
3. Pain
4. Hypothermia
5. Head and neck soft tissue edema

Postoperative Pain Intensity Moderately severe.

Postoperative Pain Control Epidural, PCA, routine parenteral.

Postoperative Tests HCT, CXR, and ECG often done.

SURGICAL PROCEDURE Organ Harvest (Brain Dead Patient)

The ideal donor is a previously healthy individual who has suffered isolated brain death. Contraindications to organ donation are advanced age, septicemia, most malignancies, and transmissible diseases not treatable with antibiotics.

Objective Retrieval of organs for transplantation.

Position Supine, with arms tucked in at the sides to facilitate access to thorax and abdomen.

Exposure Neck to pubis.

Incision Midline incision from sternal notch to pubis.

Blood Bank Order T&C 4 units PRBCs. Donor may require transfusions.

Estimated Blood Loss 1000 ml.

Preoperative Studies Confirmation of brain death. HCT, electrolytes, coagulation profile. Exact confirmation of brain death depends on country, state, region, and hospital policies. Medical definition of death is brainstem death. Diagnosis of brain death is based on the following criteria:
1. Complete unresponsiveness to stimuli. Lack of response to gag reflex, corneal reflex, pupillary reflex, apnea test for 10 minutes, atropine.
2. Known cause of death not related to toxic-metabolic causes or hypothermia.
3. Correlation with electroencephalogram, brainstem auditory evoked potentials, CT scan with contrast, angiography. These tests generally not considered essential.
4. Declaration by physician, typically neurologist, not transplant surgeon.

Anesthetic Choices No anesthetic needed since patient is unresponsive. Some spinal reflexes may be intact. Relaxants are generally administered to prevent uncoordinated reflex body movements.

Invasive Monitoring Arterial line, CVC.

Aspiration Precautions Patient already intubated.

Queries for Surgeon Which organs being harvested? Dopamine to be used? Dopamine may deplete norepinephrine stores in donor heart. Time of heparin administration is usually immediately before harvesting of heart.

Estimated Surgical Time 2 to 4 hours.

➤ **Anesthetic Considerations**
1. **Hemodynamic Instability**
   Donors develop cardiovascular instability shortly after brain death (within 24 to 48 hours).
2. **Coagulopathy**

Coagulopathy follows release of fibrinolytic substances from the brain and elsewhere.

3. **Diabetes Insipidus**

Diabetes insipidus common: lack of antidiuretic hormone (ADH) release from the posterior pituitary. Complications of diabetes insipidus include hypovolemia, hypokalemia, hypernatremia, hyperosmolality, hypocalcemia. If urine output is greater than 300–500 ml/h, administer vasopressin.

4. **Poikilothermy**

Due to loss of hypothalamic function. Invoke measures to maintain core temperature above 33° C to prevent hypothermia-induced arrhythmias and coagulopathy.

5. **Blood Loss**

Major blood loss may require transfusions to preserve organ function before harvesting.

6. **Vasopressor Support**

With loss of the brainstem and the vagus nerve, bradycardias are no longer responsive to atropine. Use direct or indirect catecholamines to treat bradyarrhythmias.

7. **Oliguria**

Oliguria is common and may be consequent to hypotension, hypovolemia, rhabdomyolysis. Treat oliguria with optimization of hemodynamics, fluid administration, furosemide, mannitol, or both.

8. **Electrolyte Abnormalities**

Electrolyte abnormalities are common (Na^+, K^+, Cl^-, Ca^{2+}).

Intraoperative Hazards

1. Hypotension.
2. Difficult resuscitation in the event of cardiac arrest.
3. Major blood loss.
4. Coagulopathy.
5. Patient's movements from spinal reflexes are unnerving to nonmedical staff.

SURGICAL PROCEDURE Pancreatic Surgery

Objective

1. *Excisional debridement* of necrotic pancreas is often the quickest way to recovery. Because the tail of the pancreas is close to the spleen, splenectomy is often inevitable.
2. *Marsupialization* of fibrous-walled pseudocyst cavity (containing tissue products digested by pancreatic enzymes) into the stomach, duodenum, or a Roux-en-Y loop of small bowel. Marsupialization relieves most pseudocyst problems.
3. *Decompression* of blocked and dilated duct of Wirsung for relief of pain and to help preserve parenchymal function in chronic pancreatitis when ducts are amenable to surgical opening. Occasionally done for duct blocked by cancer (known colloquially as Puestow, Thal, or Partington operation).

Position   Supine, left arm abducted.

Exposure   Nipples to intraumbilical region; nipples to pubis.

Incision   Midline, oblique transverse, or bilateral subcostal.

Blood Bank Order   4 units PRBCs.

Estimated Blood Loss   500 ml. May be massive if from accidental injury to spleen.

Preoperative Studies   HCT, coagulation profile, electrolytes, BUN, glucose, Ca, PO_4, albumin, CXR, and ECG; ABGs optional. Patients with pancreatic disease often have multiorgan disease.

Anesthetic Choices   General; epidural and general.

Invasive Monitoring   Arterial line, Foley; CVC and pulmonary artery catheter optional. Chemistry for glucose monitoring.

Airway Considerations   Routine.

Aspiration Precautions   Use because of GI obstruction or ileus.

Estimated Surgical Time   3 to 6 hours average.

➤ **Anesthetic Considerations**
1. **Preoperative Evaluation**
   Attention to multiorgan dysfunction, glucose intolerance, malnutrition, and underlying cause of pancreatic disease (e.g., alcohol abuse).
2. **Anesthetic Problems**
   Risk of lengthy procedure, hypothermia, abdominal distention with pancreatic phlegmon, and appreciable third space and blood losses. Limit N_2O and take care with positioning. Septic behavior requires invasive monitoring and optimization of hemodynamics and urine output.
3. **Anesthetic Management**
   a. Proper setup (large-bore IVs, fluid warmer, availability of blood, monitoring transducers, etc.)
   b. Conventional rapid sequence or modified rapid sequence induction after placement of proper monitoring. Amount of anesthetic administered may have to be limited in severely ill patient.
   c. *Maintenance:* Inhalation, narcotic, or epidural anesthetic or any combination of these. Give special consideration to anesthetic problems listed above.

Intraoperative Hazards
1. Multiple organ dysfunction syndrome (MODS) involving unstable hemodynamics, acute renal failure, DIC from systemic inflammatory response syndrome (SIRS), and respiratory failure from adult respiratory distress syndrome.
2. Surgical complications: splenic or vascular injury causing massive blood loss; pneumothorax from subdiaphragmatic surgical manipulation; and others such as bowel injury.

Postoperative Management   PACU; ICU often required.

Postoperative Pain Intensity   Severe; many patients have been receiving high-dose narcotics for a long time and thus have high narcotic tolerance.

Postoperative Pain Control   Epidural ideal if no major contraindications to it; IV narcotics are routine.

SURGICAL PROCEDURE   Parathyroid Excision

Primary hyperparathyroidism is due to adenoma, hyperplasia, carcinoma, or a nonparathyroid tumor producing parathyroid-like substance. *Secondary hyperparathyroidism* often is associated with renal disease. Hyperparathyroidism is associated with hypercalcemia and hypomagnesemia. Hypercalcemia may effect renal damage (with hypertension), mental status changes, musculoskeletal abnormalities (weakness), GI disease (ulcers, pancreatitis), and ECG conduction abnormalities (short QT interval).

Objective   Removal of hyperactive parathyroid (parathyroid adenoma) without compromising normal glands.

Position   Same as thyroid. Neck extension poorly tolerated in those with rheumatoid arthritis and in the elderly with basilar artery insufficiency.

Exposure   Chin to nipples.

Incision   Transverse on neck.

Blood Bank Order   None.

Estimated Blood Loss   Less than 100 ml.

Preoperative Studies   HCT, coagulation profile, electrolytes, BUN, creatinine, glucose, Ca^{2+}, PO_4, albumin, CXR, ECG. Treat hypercalcemia preoperatively if patient has symptoms.

Anesthetic Choices   General; or local with sedation. Spontaneous ventilation allows better assessment of airway patency and depth of anesthesia. Length of procedure can make this problematic. Armored endotracheal tube recommended.

Invasive Monitoring   Ordinarily none, but use CVC and Foley if patient is in hypercalcemic crisis. Serial calcium can be obtained by venipuncture.

Airway Considerations   Yes. Large tumor may obstruct trachea.

Aspiration Precautions   None unless an emergency procedure or patient is at risk of gastric reflux.

Queries for Surgeon
1. Superior laryngeal nerve stimulation?
2. Reimplantation of gland in arm?
3. Mediastinal exploration for ectopic parathyroid gland?

Estimated Surgical Time   Time can be 2 to 6 hours. At least two glands are sampled to make sure disease is not hyperplasia.

➤ ### Anesthetic Considerations
1. Limited access to face.
2. Risk of endotracheal tube's kinking or disconnecting.
3. Positioning to prevent facial or eye injuries.
4. Metabolic problems.
5. Surgeon may want to stimulate superior laryngeal nerve. Maintain at least one twitch in train-of-four.
6. Confirm vocal cord function by laryngoscopy during extubation.

Intraoperative Hazards
1. Hyperthermia due to complete draping and little exposure
2. Face and eye injury from tubes, instruments, or surgeons
3. Orotracheal tube's kinking and disconnecting
4. Pneumothorax

Postoperative Problems
1. Airway compromise by hematoma
2. Recurrent laryngeal nerve injury
3. Rebound hypocalcemia (due to "hungry bones") with tetany and cord spasm
4. Laryngeal edema or tracheomalacia.
Monitor serum calcium and replace calcium intravenously as needed. Initially may treat laryngeal edema with nebulized racemic epinephrine.

Postoperative Pain Control   Parenteral day of surgery; oral or none thereafter.

Postoperative Tests   Serum calcium, phosphate, albumin.

SURGICAL PROCEDURE   Pilonidal Cyst or Sinus Excision

Objective   Removal of sinus tracts and cystic areas.

Position   Prone, jackknife.

Exposure   Lower back to midthigh.

Incision   Over sacrum and coccyx.

Blood Bank Order   None.

Estimated Blood Loss   Minimal.

Preoperative Studies   Routine.

Anesthetic Choices   General, spinal, lumbar or epidural, or local. Spinal with hypobaric tetracaine or lidocaine may be performed with patient in jackknife position. If pilonidal cyst is infected, regional lumbar technique is contraindicated because of proximity of infection and site of needle insertion.

Invasive Monitoring   None.

Airway Considerations   Routine.

Aspiration Precautions   None unless an emergency procedure or patient is at risk of gastric reflux.

Estimated Surgical Time   30 to 60 minutes.

➤ **Anesthetic Considerations**
Similar to those for hemorrhoidectomy:
1. Short procedure.
2. Generally healthy patients.
3. Safe positioning.
4. Hazard of accidental extubation in prone position.
5. Caveat regarding overdistension of bladder holds for men with pilonidal sinuses also.

Postoperative Pain Intensity   Mild to moderate.

Postoperative Pain Control   Parenteral or oral narcotics.

SURGICAL PROCEDURE   Portasystemic Shunt Procedures

Includes portacaval shunt, mesocaval shunt, and proximal and distal splenorenal shunts. Not commonly used since advent of transinternal jugular portasystemic shunt (TIPSS). Many authorities, without proof, regard distal splenorenal shunt as being superior to other portasystemic shunting procedures, because of the associated low risk of postoperative hepatic failure and encephalopathy. This is a patient population with end-stage chronic liver disease resulting in cirrhosis, portal hypertension, esophageal varices, ascites, encephalopathy, coagulopathy, and low albumin. The problems with portasystemic shunting procedures are
1. A reduction in hepatic blood flow that may be deleterious to the liver itself
2. The shunting of mesenteric blood (nonfiltration of toxins by the liver) directly into the systemic circulation
Child's classification of patients as A, B, or C correlates with their prognosis. Emergency procedures have a high mortality rate.

Objectives
1. To decrease high splanchnic pressure secondary to an intrahepatic or extrahepatic blockage and to decompress engorged collateral veins (high pressure splanchnic vein drains into low pressure systemic vein).

2. To reduce portal hypertension and collateral blood flow in order to decrease variceal bleeding.

Position   Supine with roll under right flank. Right arm suspended.

Exposure   Abdomen, lower thorax, and flank.

Incision   Long right subcostal or midline abdominal.

Blood Bank Order   T&C 6 units PRBCs, FFP, cryoprecipitate, and platelets as deemed necessary by patient's coagulopathy. Blood salvaging technique recommended (e.g., autotransfuser).

Estimated Blood Loss   600 to 1000 ml. May be massive.

Preoperative Studies   CBC, coagulation profile (PT, PTT, platelets), electrolytes, BUN, creatinine, glucose, alkaline phosphatase, AST, ALT, ammonia, albumin, LDH, amylase, CXR, ECG. Studies of nutritional status, coagulation, and hepatic, renal, and pulmonary functions indicated. Albumin and PT and bilirubin levels regarded as most important indicators of postoperative prognosis.

Preoperative Medications   Vitamin K given several days before surgery in consideration of coagulopathy. Steroid stress doses are given if patient has received steroids for hepatitis. Antacids or metoclopramide or both are given. Avoid sedatives unless patient is receiving benzodiazepine for alcohol withdrawal.

Anesthetic Choices   General; epidural optional if no contraindications to epidural (namely coagulopathy).

Invasive Monitoring   Arterial line, CVC, and Foley; pulmonary artery catheter optional. Poor splanchnic flow, moderate blood loss, multiple organ dysfunction (renal, CNS, hematologic), and major fluid shifts require close monitoring.

Airway Considerations   Routine oral endotracheal tube (OETT).

Aspiration Precautions   Full aspiration precautions. Regurgitation and aspiration potential with ascites, advanced encephalopathy, and GI bleeding. Therefore, awake, rapid sequence or modified rapid sequence intubation is indicated.

Estimated Surgical Time   3 to 6 hours.

▶ **Anesthetic Considerations**
 1. **Preoperative Evaluation**
     a. Underlying cause. End-stage liver disease from major organ involvement. For example, patient may have alcoholic cirrhosis with associated multiorgan disease or α-1 antitrypsin deficiency with associated pulmonary disease.
     b. Associated medical conditions. Cirrhosis may be associated with
         (1) Pulmonary disease: oxygen desaturation when erect (orthodeoxia), platypnea, pulmonary shunts, effusions.

     (2) Cardiac alterations: high cardiac output, possible associated cardiomyopathy.

     (3) Hematologic problems: thrombocytopenia, coagulopathy, anemia, vitamin A deficiency.

     (4) Renal disease: susceptibility to hepatorenal syndrome.

     (5) CNS system: encephalopathy with increased sensitivity to anesthetics.

     (6) Ascites: control and relieve ascites preoperatively if possible.

  c. Perioperative antibiotic requirements.

  d. Protection of hospital personnel against viral hepatitis.

2. Intraoperative Management

Because placing a portasystemic shunt is a major procedure requiring a large incision, major fluid shifts, rapid loss of ascites, and third space and blood losses can be expected.

  a. Maintenance of good hemodynamics is most important in preventing deterioration of hepatic function in already tenuous circulation and hepatorenal syndrome.

  b. Major determinants of hepatic blood flow:

     (1) Type of procedure.

     (2) Hemodynamics.

     (3) Ventilation: decreased P_{CO_2} and alterations in CO_2 homeostasis (e.g., hypocapnia) may decrease hepatic circulation (maintenance of normocapnia).

     (4) Anesthetic drugs.

  c. Large-bore IV access. Prevention of hypothermia with major fluid or blood product requirements.

  d. Altered pharmacodynamics. Increased sensitivity to CNS depressants in end-stage liver disease. Chronic alcoholic nonencephalopathic patient may have a tolerance requiring large doses of thiopental for induction.

  e. Altered pharmacokinetics. Impaired hepatic clearance of drugs increases volume of distribution of most drugs and increases relaxant requirements; often renal clearance impaired also. Inhalation anesthetic technique in patients with major liver disease is rational choice; twitch monitor would be useful; unpredictable relaxant dosage requirement.

  f. Coagulopathy considerations.

     (1) Monitor intraoperative coagulation studies (e.g., platelets, PT, PTT, thromboelastogram).

     (2) Avoid regional technique or subclavian CVC in severe coagulopathy.

  g. Impaired glucose homeostasis. Monitor serum glucose levels.

  h. *Maintenance:* Isoflurane reduces hepatic blood flow less than halothane does. Inhalation or IV narcotic technique is acceptable.

  i. *Emergence.* Consider postoperative overnight endotracheal intubation until patient is stable.

Intraoperative Hazards

1. Air embolism

2. Hypovolemia

3. Massive blood loss

4. Renal shut down

5. Hypoglycemia

6. Poor gas exchange
7. Electrolyte abnormalities
8. Laceration of portal vein or its tributaries

Postoperative Management   ICU.

Postoperative Problems
1. Encephalopathy common with most portasystemic shunt procedures
2. Hepatic failure
3. Infection
4. Bleeding and coagulopathy
5. Renal failure (hepatorenal syndrome)
6. Hypothermia

Postoperative Pain Intensity   Severe.

Postoperative Pain Control   Epidural, PCA, routine IV.

Postoperative Tests   Complete routine biochemistries and hematology studies, ECG, CXR.

SURGICAL PROCEDURE   Thyroid Resection

Objective   Removal of malignant or hyperactive thyroid nodule.

Position   Supine, with neck extended (by inflated bag under shoulders after intubation). Arms at sides.

Exposure   Chin to nipples.

Incision   Transverse neck incision.

Blood Bank Order   T&S.

Estimated Blood Loss   Less than 100 ml.

Preoperative Studies   Routine plus thyroid function tests. May require treatment for hyperthyroidism unless an emergency procedure. Large goiter can impinge on airway. Get flow-volume loops, bronchoscopy, tracheal tomograms to assess trachea if upper airway obstruction suspected.

Anesthetic Choices   General anesthesia; cervical epidural a possible alternative.

Invasive Monitoring   None.

Airway Considerations   May have intrathoracic or extrathoracic tracheal compression. With demonstrated or suspected airway compromise, intubate while preserving spontaneous ventilation.

Aspiration Precautions   Not necessary unless an emergency procedure or patient is at risk of gastric reflux.

Queries for Surgeon   Unilateral or bilateral procedure?

Estimated Surgical Time   Variable; 2 hours.

➤ **Anesthetic Considerations**
  1. **Preoperative Evaluation and Optimization**
     Acute treatment of thyrotoxic storm: IV propranolol, sodium iodide IV (unless patient is pregnant), and steroids.
  2. **Anesthetic Problems**
     a. Limited view of patient except top of head
     b. Face and eye injury from equipment
     c. Extubation or disconnection under drapes
     d. Stimulation intensity variable, greatest during dissection near trachea
     e. Avoid neck lines
     f. Risk of thyroid storm
     g. Air embolism, carotid sinus stimulation
     h. Injury to superior or recurrent laryngeal nerves (RLN). Unilateral complete RLN injury causes hoarseness of voice and paramedian position of involved cord. Most dangerous situation is that in which there is bilateral partial damage to the RLN, leaving the adductor fibers unopposed and complete airway obstruction. Laryngoscopy or bronchoscopy may be done at end of procedure with patient under deep anesthesia to verify vocal cord function.

Postoperative Problems   Respiratory compromise due to
  1. Airway problems: extrinsic tracheal hematoma, RLN injury, tracheomalacia, hypocalcemic laryngeal tetany. If hematoma compromises airway, open the wound immediately, as endotracheal intubation may be difficult until hematoma is relieved. Hypocalcemia would be due to iatrogenic, inadvertent parathyroidectomy.
  2. Thoracic problems: pneumothorax.

Postoperative Pain Intensity   Mild.

Postoperative Pain Control   Parenteral narcotics to oral narcotics day 1 after surgery.

Postoperative Tests   Thyroid function tests, Ca^{2+}, PO_4, CXR.

SURGICAL PROCEDURE   Tracheostomy

Objective   Bypass nasopharynx and oropharynx. Reasons for tracheostomy include prospect of prolonged intubation, upper airway obstruction (trauma, tumor), and airway protection from chronic aspiration.

Position   Supine with neck extended. Arms tucked at side.

Exposure   Neck and upper thorax.

Incision   Small, between thyroid isthmus and sternal notch.

Blood Bank Order   T&S.

Estimated Blood Loss   None.

Preoperative Studies   Routine and as dictated by underlying disease. May require evaluation of upper airway or pulmonary status.

Anesthetic Choices   General with oral or nasal endotracheal intubation (ETT) or local anesthetic. General anesthesia is appropriate for patients who are already intubated. Nonintubated patients with upper-airway or oral abnormalities may be safely approached with local anesthesia.

Invasive Monitoring   None.

Airway Considerations   Close cooperation between surgeon and anesthesiologist needed.

Aspiration Precautions   Depend on underlying condition but are necessary in an emergency procedure or if patient is at risk of gastric reflux.

Estimated Surgical Time   30 minutes to 1 hour.

➤ **Anesthetic Considerations**
1. **Preoperative Evaluation**
   a. Routine assessment including airway evaluation and risk of aspiration.
   b. Selection of general or local anesthesia depends on such factors as patient cooperation, patient preference, and ease of orotracheal intubation.
2. **Anesthetic Problems**
   a. Often severely debilitated patient population.
   b. Potential for loss of airway control during procedure.
   c. Patient's movement if he or she is not paralyzed.
   d. Muscle relaxants: *advantage* is no patient movement or agitation. *Disadvantage* is absence of spontaneous ventilation in event of loss of surgical airway.
3. **Anesthetic Management**
   a. Tailor anesthesia for short procedure.
   b. 100% oxygen in event of lost airway.
   c. After surgeon has made tracheal incision and is ready to insert tracheostomy tube, remove the OETT slowly while keeping it just below the glottis. Close coordination with surgeon is essential at this step.
   d. Confirm bilateral breath sounds and $ETCO_2$ immediately after tracheostomy is placed in trachea.
   e. With local anesthetic technique, administration of rapid acting IV agents (e.g., thiopental, propofol, lidocaine) may be required to control coughing as soon as tracheostomy tube placement is confirmed.

Intraoperative Hazards
1. Difficult orotracheal intubation

2. Loss of airway in paralyzed patient
3. Creation of false passage with tracheostomy tube
4. Bleeding obscuring control of airway
5. Sudden patient movement
6. Arrhythmia

Postoperative Problems
1. Bleeding
2. Pneumothorax
3. Pneumomediastinum
4. Accidental extubation. Accidental extubation of a fresh tracheostomy is a serious problem. Orotracheal intubation is generally recommended unless stoma is open and sutures around stoma are available for traction during reinsertion. There is a risk of tracheal collapse, creation of a false passage, or bleeding during tracheostomy reinsertion.

Postoperative Pain Intensity   Minimal.

Postoperative Pain Control   Routine.

Postoperative Tests   CXR to confirm proper tracheostomy placement and to rule out pneumothorax.

SURGICAL PROCEDURE   Trauma

Objective   Surgery for the trauma patient; 50% of trauma-related deaths occur at the scene of the accident; 30% of trauma-related deaths occur within 3 hours of the accident, mostly from exsanguination and hypoxia (in the "golden" initial hours, resuscitation may save the life); 20% of trauma-related deaths occur late in the day or weeks following, mostly from sepsis or multiorgan failure.

Blood Bank Order   The following products are ordered as indicated and, most importantly, in anticipation of need: fresh whole blood, PRBCs, platelets, FFP, cryoprecipitate, colloids (i.e., albumin or hetastarch). In trauma situations, send blood out for crossmatching as soon as possible (as soon as a good IV is established). Administer crystalloids through large-bore IV until blood products are available. Order blood products as needed. Reassess availability of blood continuously. Avoid being caught with no blood products. Consider blood salvage systems. Avoid venous access and fluid administration distal to area of trauma (e.g., fluid administration via lower extremity venous access in patient with abdominal or pelvic injuries). In massive transfusion (i.e., >10 units of blood or one blood volume replacement), use of fresh whole blood (<6 hours old) is indicated because of its volume and coagulation benefits. However, many institutions do not have fresh whole blood available. The optimal source of RBCs is fully typed and crossmatched blood, but it requires 45 minutes to prepare. Second choice would be blood typed and screened. Third, simply typed blood (requires 5 minutes for blood bank to prepare). Lastly, universal donor packed cells (O-positive or O-negative for men and O-negative for women). Platelets are administered in massive transfusions if indicated clinically by patient's bleeding diathesis (e.g., oozing or "medical bleeding") or by laboratory studies (administer platelets in massive transfusions or major surgery to keep platelet count over 75,000). Administer fresh frozen plasma if indicated clinically by a bleeding diathesis or by laboratory studies (elevated PT, PTT, or ACT is thought to be due to coagulation factor deficiency). Cryoprecipitate primarily contains factors I and VIII. Administer all blood products through blood macrofilters. Use microfilters only optionally in RBC transfusions; calcium (1 CaCl every 5 units of blood) is given to prevent hemodynamic effects of hypocalcemia only if >1 unit blood is administered every 3 to 5 minutes; HCT may not reflect blood loss, as time is needed for hemodilution to occur.

Preoperative Studies   CBC, electrolytes, Ca^{2+}, Mg, BUN, creatinine, glucose, CPK, LFTs, ABGs, crossmatch, urine, myoglobin, toxicology screen (including barbiturates, benzodiazepines, alcohol, cocaine, narcotics, tricyclic antidepressants), CXR, ECG, cervical spine x-rays. Preoperative laboratory studies are sent for as indicated and if time permits.

Anesthetic Choices   General, regional, or local (if possible). Regional anesthesia is suitable in surgery on the extremities in a cooperative patient as long as there is no hemodynamic, respiratory, or neurologic compromise and no significant coagulopathy (especially for epidurals). General anesthesia may consist merely of paralysis, oxygen, and endotracheal intubation (ETI) in a severely hypovolemic and hypotensive patient who would be unable to tolerate any anesthetic. Scopolamine may be the only sedative given initially. Ketamine (1–2 mg/kg) or etomidate (0.2–0.3 mg/kg) are good induction alternatives to thiopental in a somewhat hemodynamically compromised patient. As patient is resuscitated, anesthetics such as inhalation agents, narcotics, and benzodiazepines are titrated.

Invasive Monitoring   In severe trauma, in addition to routine monitoring, intraoperative monitoring consists of arterial line, CVC, and Foley.
1. Arterial line benefits: continuous BP monitoring; assessment of fluid status (i.e., respiratory variations, pulse pressure, width of curve); and availability of ABGs. Automated cuff readings in severe hypovolemia may be fallacious, as patient moves erratically.
2. CVC is indicated for fluid status assessment, venous access, rapid drug administration, and possible conversion to a pulmonary artery catheter (PAC).
3. Foley is inserted only if there is no blood at the urethral meatus. It is most useful for fluid management, assessment of renal perfusion, and to check for myoglobinuria and hemoglobinuria.
4. PAC generally is not necessary unless cardiovascular assessment is complicated by problems such as valvular heart disease, myocardial dysfunction, or pulmonary hypertension.
5. Intracranial pressure (ICP) monitoring is indicated in major head trauma (clinically or by CT scan) to detect and manage worsening intracranial bleeding or cerebral edema in patient who is about to undergo prolonged general anesthetic.

Airway Considerations
1. Stabilize cervical spine or rule out cervical spine injury before manipulating airway or transporting patient.

2. Indications for surgical airway (cricothyrotomy or transtracheal ventilation) are inability to orally or nasally intubate and significant facial injuries.
3. Nasal intubation is contraindicated in suspected basal skull fractures ("raccoon eyes" or "battle sign"), facial injuries, Lefort's II and III facial fractures, and major coagulopathy. Otherwise, it is useful in agitated patient because patient cooperation not required. Often used in setting outside of OR (e.g., emergency room).
4. Fiberoptic intubations rarely are used in emergency setting.

Aspiration Precautions Trauma patients considered to have full stomachs. Consequently, ETI should be performed either in awake patient or after rapid sequence or modified rapid sequence induction. Superior laryngeal and transtracheal nerve blocks are relatively contraindicated because they increase risk of aspiration. Metoclopramide needs to be administered 30–60 minutes before induction; clear antacids may be given 15 minutes before induction, or H_2-blockers may be given prophylactically 30–60 minutes before induction.

➤ **Anesthetic Considerations**
Major considerations are cervical spine, airway, hemodynamics, fluid resuscitation, temperature, coagulopathy, multiorgan system involvement (CNS, pulmonary, cardiac, visceral, renal, and musculoskeletal injuries), and metabolic considerations. Diagnosis is based on primary and secondary assessment. Primary assessment is ABCs. Secondary assessment is a more complete history and physical examination and review of available laboratory tests.

1. **Anesthetic Technique**
Make sure airway is not difficult to intubate before induction of paralysis; remember full stomach considerations. Beware of thiopental's deleterious hemodynamic effects: hypovolemia, cardiac depression, vasodilatation, and removal of sympathetic stimulation, which is accentuated by decreased venous return after positive pressure ventilation. Succinylcholine provides fastest onset of paralysis for rapid sequence intubation. As an induction agent, ketamine or etomidate may produce less hypotension than thiopental will. Anesthetic maintenance requirements may vary significantly as stability of patient changes. Avoid N_2O if patient requires high FiO_2 or if has closed airspace (e.g., pneumothorax); otherwise N_2O may be used. Keep patient intubated at end of surgery if he or she is hemodynamically unstable, has pulmonary disease, is hypothermic, and is not protecting airway and for expected major fluid shifts after massive resuscitation.

2. **Multiorgan System Involvement**
Patients may have multiorgan system involvement (e.g., lung contusion, cardiac contusion, CNS injury, multiple bone fractures) or may develop multisystem failure secondarily (adult respiratory distress syndrome, disseminated intravascular coagulation, acute renal failure, cerebral edema, sepsis).
   a. Protect kidneys from crush injury–induced rhabdomyolysis with aggressive fluid management and mannitol (0.25–2.0 g/kg), plus furosemide if indicated.
   b. Consider aortic arch involvement in rapid deceleration injuries, widened mediastinum, sternal, clavicular, or 1st or 2nd rib fractures, lateral tracheal shift, and blunting of aortic knob. Standard for diagnosis is arch aortogram.

3. **Metabolic**

Acid-base abnormalities most often from hypotensive lactic acidosis or hyperchloremic metabolic acidosis. Consider diabetic ketoacidosis and drug-related acidosis (e.g., methanol, alcohol, salicylates); also hypoglycemia, which often is overlooked in the comatose patient. Hypocalcemia and hyperkalemia occur in rapid massive transfusions (>150 ml/min of blood.)

4. **Miscellaneous**

Has patient received tetanus toxoid? Antibiotics for open wounds? Is patient pregnant? Is patient wearing contact lenses? Has family been notified?

Intraoperative Hazards Always return to basics when patient deteriorates. First things first: ABCs. Consider oxygenation, ventilation, hemodynamics, metabolism, drugs, and anesthetics (or lack of) for any problems that arise perioperatively (e.g., hypotension, hypertension, hypoxemia, shortness of breath, bradycardia, tachycardia, agitation).

Postoperative Problems Depend on type of injury.

Postoperative Pain Control Typically managed with IV narcotics in ICU.

SURGICAL PROCEDURE Truncal Vagotomy

Objective Reduce gastric acid secretion. Severence of two main vagal trunks, removing stimuli to entire stomach. Always combined with pyloroplasty. "Highly selective" vagotomy (HSV) preserves gastric antral motility; therefore does not require pyloroplasty but is associated with a high rate of recurrence of excessive gastric acid secretion. However, with the advent of potent H_2-receptor blockers and proton pump inhibitors, the need for HSV is diminishing.

Position Supine, left arm extended.

Exposure Upper abdomen.

Incision Midline.

Blood Bank Order T&S.

Estimated Blood Loss Less than 300 ml.

Preoperative Studies Routine plus at least HCT for all patients with a bleeding diathesis (peptic ulcer disease [PUD]).

Anesthetic Choices General; epidural optional.

Invasive Monitoring None.

Airway Considerations Routine.

Aspiration Precautions   Present for upper GI bleeding, gastric-outlet obstruction, and emergency procedures.

Estimated Surgical Time   Less than 2 hours.

➤ **Anesthetic Considerations**
1. **Preoperative Evaluation and Optimization**
   Routine; plus pay special attention to underlying cause of PUD (e.g., alcohol, NSAID), hemodynamic status if associated with upper GI bleed, and associated medical problems.
2. **Anesthetic Concerns**
   a. Related to preoperative problems
   b. Possible full stomach
   c. Relatively short procedure
   d. Muscle relaxation preferable for surgical exposure
   e. Extubation period
3. **Intraoperative Hazards**
   a. Splenic injury
   b. Bleeding
   c. Vagal reactions

Postoperative Pain Control   Epidural, PCA, intercostal blocks, routine.

SUGGESTED READINGS
Trauma
Malt RA. The Practice of Surgery. Philadelphia: W.B. Saunders, 1993.
Matjasko MJ, Shin B. Anesthesia and Trauma. In Problems in Anesthesia. Philadelphia: J.B. Lippincott, vol 4, Sept 1990.
Steve J, Grande C. Trauma Anesthesiology. Baltimore: Williams & Wilkins, 1991.

Liver Transplantation
Carmichael FJ, Lindop MJ, Farman JV. Anesthesia for Hepatic Transplantation: Cardiovascular and Metabolic Alterations and Their Management. Anesth Analg 64:108, 1985.
Firestone L, Firestone S. Anesthesia for Organ Transplantation. In Clinical Anaesthesia. Philadelphia: J.B. Lippincott, 1992.
Yoogoo K. Hepatic Transplantation. In Anesthesiology Clinics of North America. Philadelphia: W.B. Saunders, vol 7, Sept 1989.

CHAPTER 5

ELECTROCONVULSIVE THERAPY AND EYE SURGERY

SURGICAL PROCEDURE Electroconvulsive Therapy (ECT)

Objective Electrical induction of seizure. Duration of recommended seizure activity for therapeutic effectiveness is >30 seconds. Indication for ECT is severe depression unresponsive to pharmacologic therapy.

Preoperative Studies Routine.

Preoperative Medication Atropine or labetolol sometimes used to blunt cardiac response.

Anesthetic Choices General anesthesia with mask.

➤ **Anesthetic Considerations**
1. **Preoperative Evaluation and Contraindications**
   Routine evaluation plus special considerations to cardiovascular diseases and psychotropic drugs. Generally not possible to discontinue medications, e.g., MAO inhibitors.
   a. Major drug interactions
      (1) Tricyclic antidepressants increase effect of direct-acting sympathomimetics up to tenfold.
      (2) MAO inhibitors in concert with indirect-acting sympathomimetics can induce a hypertensive crisis.
      (3) MAO inhibitors used with direct-acting sympathomimetics, also may elicit a hypertensive response, though less severe
      (4) MAO inhibitors may interact with narcotics to produce an excitatory or depressive reaction. Consequently, meperidine is contraindicated. Other narcotics, if used at all, should be titrated initially in ¼ to ⅓ the usual dose.
   b. *Contraindications:* Strong contraindications to ECT are patients with an intracranial mass lesion, cerebrovascular anomalies, elevated intracranial pressure, or a recent myocardial infarction.
2. **Anesthetic Goals**
   a. Provide lack of awareness, since electrical shocks may not produce seizure activity.

89

b. Prevent bodily injury during seizure.
c. Protect mouth and tongue with bite-block.
d. Ensure rapid recovery.
e. Prevent and treat side-effects, especially cardiovascular and respiratory.

3. Anesthetic Technique
a. Full preoperative evaluation.
b. Premedication with atropine or labetolol or Esmolol administered immediately before induction (1.0–1.5 mg/kg) sometimes is used to blunt cardiac response.
c. Routine monitoring and IV access established.
d. Induction provided with short duration agent such as methohexital 0.6–1.0 mg/kg (reduces seizure threshold), with pentothal 1.5–2.5 mg/kg (increases seizure threshold; therefore limit dose), or with propofol 1.0–1.5 mg/kg (has no reported effects on seizure threshold) followed by succinylcholine 0.5 mg/kg.
e. Place tongue protector.
f. Induce seizure by ECT.
g. Oxygenate by mask and allow patient to awaken spontaneously.

4. Procedure-related Events
Immediately after the electroshock (assuming successful seizure induction) there is a parasympathetic-sympathetic activation sequence that initiates a vagal discharge that lasts up to 20 seconds, followed by a sympathetic discharge for approximately 1 minute, followed by a recovery period. Most frequent ECG abnormalities: atrial arrhythmias, nodal rhythm, premature ventricular contractions, sinus bradycardia, and sinus tachycardia. Most patients do not require any treatment for these otherwise alarming rhythms, as the rhythm disturbances are almost always short lived.

SURGICAL PROCEDURE Eye Surgery

Includes cataract, scleral buckle, strabismus, and open globe procedures.

Objectives
1. *Cataract:* Removal of opacified lens.
2. *Scleral buckle:* Surgical management of retinal detachment.
3. *Strabismus:* Surgical correction of ocular deviation on ocular muscles.
4. *Open globe:* Removal of foreign body and closure of open globe, generally the result of trauma.

Position Supine.

Estimated Blood Loss None.

Preoperative Laboratory Studies Routine.

Anesthetic Choices General anesthesia with oral endotracheal tube (OETT); or retrobulbar block with or without IV sedation.

Invasive Monitoring   None.

Aspiration Precautions   Necessary precautions with open globe procedures because of full stomach status.

Queries for Surgeon   Open globe? Regional or general anesthesia?

Estimated Surgical Time   1 to 2 hours.

➤ **Anesthetic Considerations**
Generally, ocular procedures involve only low-level stimulation and consequently carry low risk. Children require general anesthesia for all procedures.

1. **Immobile Eye (Akinesis)**
   Achieved by retrobulbar block or by providing adequate depth of general anesthesia with or without use of a muscle relaxant.

2. **Oculocardiac Reflex**
   Trigeminovagal reflex prevention and treatment: ensure adequate oxygenation, hemodynamics, and depth of anesthesia. First ask surgeon to stop stimulation transiently; then use IV atropine or infiltrate rectus muscles with a local anesthetic or do both.

3. **Nausea and Vomiting**
   High incidence of postoperative emesis, especially in strabismus procedures. Prevention and treatment with antiemetics, e.g., droperidol (25–70 µg/kg), and avoidance of N_2O may be of benefit.

4. **Intraocular Pressure (IOP) Considerations**
   When IOP considerations are applicable, e.g., open globe procedures, aim to provide smooth anesthesia and BP control. Prevent straining, minimize increases in venous pressure, and provide adequate ventilation and oxygenation for PCO_2 and PaO_2 control. Avoid use of ketamine. Consider deep extubation on emergence.

5. **Associated Medical Problems**
   Elderly are easily confused and often have multiple associated medical conditions. Blind patients quite apprehensive.

6. **Patient Suitability for Retrobulbar Block**
   Patient must be able to communicate and understand and must be a good candidate for an awake surgical procedure in a claustrophobic environment under retrobulbar block.

7. **Drugs**
   Succinylcholine may cause transient and mild increases in intraocular pressure (IOP); thus it is often avoided intraoperatively with open globe procedures. However, it may be used on induction with precurarization. Ketamine is generally avoided in eye surgery; may cause nystagmus, increases in IOP, blepharospasm, and visual hallucinations. IM atropine not contraindicated in glaucoma, although probably not effective in prevention of oculocardiac reflex.

8. **Optic Drugs**
   Timolol and scopolamine have systemic effects. Anticholinesterase effect of echothiophate is prolonged (4 to 6 weeks after its discontinuation).

9. **Considerations for Specific Procedures**
   a. *Open globe in adult:* Suspect associated injuries and full stomach; aim for smooth induction; be careful with mask ventilation to avoid pressure on eye and elevations of IOP.

b. *Open globe in child:* Best managed with IV rapid-sequence induction.

c. *Strabismus:* Remote association with malignant hyperthermia.

Intraoperative Hazards   Paralysis and twitch monitoring are recommended with general anesthesia because of the following hazards:

1. Patient movement or coughing may be disastrous if surgeon is not expecting it (e.g., intraoperative cough with inadequate muscle relaxation or depth of anesthesia).
2. Oculocardiac reflex, nausea, and vomiting.
3. Patient agitation during retrobulbar block.
4. Intraocular, subarachnoid, or intravascular injection of local anesthetic during retrobulbar block. Intraocular injection can severely damage eye; subarachnoid or intravascular injection would produce loss of consciousness or seizures.
5. Perioperative hypertension.
6. Mask ventilation requires special attention.

Postoperative Management   Consists of keeping patient's head elevated 15 to 20 degrees with protective shield on eye and prophylaxis and treatment of nausea and vomiting.

Postoperative Problems   Nausea, vomiting, hypertension, and agitation.

Postoperative Pain Intensity   Mild.

Postoperative Pain Control   PO narcotics and nonnarcotics.

SUGGESTED READINGS
Electroconvulsive Therapy (ECT)
Messick J, Jr, Mackenzie RA, Nugent M. Anesthesia at Remote Locations. In Miller RD (ed), Anesthesia. New York: Churchill Livingstone, 1990.

Gaines GT, Rees DI. ECT and Anesthetic Considerations. Anesth Analg 65:1345, 1986.

Eye Surgery
Donlon J, Jr. Anesthesia and Eye, Ear, Nose & Throat Surgery. New York: Churchill Livingstone, 1990.

McGoldrick KE. Opthalmic Procedures on an Outpatient Basis. In McGoldrick KF (ed), Anesthesia for Opthalmic & Otolaryngologic Surgery. Philadelphia: W.B. Saunders, 1992.

CHAPTER 6

NEUROSURGICAL PROCEDURES

SURGICAL PROCEDURE Aneurysm, Craniotomy

Cerebral aneurysm typically is located in the circle of Willis. Cerebral aneurysm most often is diagnosed after a subarachnoid hemorrhage (SAH). Following is the Hunt and Hess Classification of Intracranial Aneurysm with SAH:

Grade   I: Asymptomatic
Grade   II: Moderate-to-severe headache or nuchal rigidity
Grade III: Mild focal deficit or mild mental depression
Grade IV: Moderate-to-severe focal (e.g., hemiparesis) or general neurologic deficit
Grade   V: Deep coma

Classic presentation of SAH is a sudden severe headache with or without meningeal irritation, focal deficit, and mental status changes.

Objective   To clip or cut aneurysm or to ligate parent vessel.

Position   Supine or lateral.

Exposure   After removal of the bone flap, much of the sphenoid ridge is removed and the dura is opened to allow dissection of the major vessels.

Incision   For middle cerebral posterior communicating and anterior communicating aneurysms the incision is generally frontotemporal, extending from in front of the ear to the forehead, with the patient's head turned partly or completely to the opposite side

Preoperative Studies   HCT, coagulation profile, electrolytes, glucose, BUN, creatinine, ECG. Patients may have extensive ECG changes related to SAH (most commonly ST and T wave abnormalities).

Preoperative Medication   Adequate sedation in patient with normal mental status. The goal of preoperative sedation is to avoid anxiety-provoked hypertension.

Blood Bank Order   T&C 3 units PRBCs to be kept available in OR.

Estimated Blood Loss   Negligible to massive.

Anesthetic Choice   General.

Invasive Monitoring   Arterial line, central venous catheter (CVC), Foley.

Airway Considerations   Oral endotracheal tube (OETT).

Aspiration Precautions   None unless an emergency procedure or patient is at risk of gastric reflux.

Queries for Surgeon   Induced hypotension? Barbiturate (7–15 mg/kg) before ligation of major feeding vessel because of its potential for brain protection?

Estimated Surgical Time   Variable. Often are prolonged, delicate procedures.

➤ **Anesthetic Considerations**
Operative exposure of the aneurysm may result in its rupture. Consequent blood loss can be explosive. Transient intraoperative hypotension is necessary to allow clipping of the aneurysm and sometimes temporary ligation of a major feeding vessel. However, because brain infarction may occur, some surgeons prefer normal to elevated blood pressure during temporary ligation of major vessel.

1. **Anesthetic Goals and Concerns**
   a. The five major perioperative hazards are bleeding, rebleeding, vasospasm, syndrome of inappropriate antidiuretic hormone (SIADH), and hydrocephalus.
   b. Goals are to prevent rupture of aneurysm perioperatively and to optimize cerebral hemodynamics.
   c. Measures to decrease intracranial pressure (ICP) are not taken, since decreasing ICP would increase transmural pressure gradient across vessel, which would increase risk of aneurysm rupture; normocapnia is maintained. Some brain shrinkage is required for exposure of cerebral blood vessels, however, so moderate hyperventilation may be required after dural opening.
   d. Smooth induction. Carefully control induction and intubation to avoid hypercapnia, hypoxia, hypertension, or hypotension.
   e. Paralysis is required to prevent patient movement and coughing. Intraoperative patient movement or coughing can be disastrous, (i.e., surgical mishap, brain herniation through craniotomy).
   f. Avoid hypertension and agitation. Have vasopressor, vasodilator (e.g., nitroprusside), and fast-acting sedative (thiopental) readily available.
   g. Avoid volume depletion to lessen risk of vasospasm.
   h. Induce transient hypotension during actual aneurysm clipping.
   i. Repair of giant aneurysms sometimes requires controlled hypotension or even circulatory arrest with profound hypothermia (15° to 18° C).
2. **Anesthetic Technique**
   a. General anesthesia typically is induced with thiopental, a narcotic such as fentanyl 5–10 µg/h or sufentanil 1–2 µg/h, vecuronium 0.1–0.2 mg/kg, and lidocaine 1 mg/kg and is maintained on vecuronium, fentanyl 1–2 µg/h or sufentanil 0.1–0.2 µg/h, N_2O, and a low-dose inhalation volatile anesthetic such as isoflurane.
   b. Maintain even-to-negative fluid balance, using 0.9% normal saline (Ringer's lactate is hypotonic).

c. *Emergence:* Extubation can be done with patient under deep anesthesia or awake. In any case, an early awakening and postoperative extubation are attempted to verify neurologic status unless the patient was severely depressed neurologically before surgery or underwent circulatory arrest during surgery. During emergence, to avoid cough and hypertension, consider use of IV lidocaine, esmolol, or propofol or any combination of these.

Intraoperative Hazards
1. *Aneurysm rupture:* Because of the risk of aneurysm rupture an arterial line, large-bore IV, 4 units of cross-matched blood, vasopressors and vasodilators should be available in the OR. Induced temporary severe hypotension may be required to allow surgeon good access to bleeding vessel. After bleeding is controlled, resuscitate with blood and fluids.
2. Patient's moving may cause an increase in ICP with herniation of brain through craniotomy site and can cause scalp laceration from pin holders or a surgical mishap.

Postoperative Management   ICU.

Postoperative Problems
1. Neurologic deficit due to surgical complication
2. Vasospasm
3. SIADH
4. Hydrocephalus
Vasospasm typically occurs between days 4 and 14 after SAH. Vasospasm occurs in 30–70% of patients after aneurysmal SAH. Vasospasm therapy includes (1) fluid hydration, (2) elevation of BP, (3) hemodilution, (4) calcium channel blockers.

SURGICAL PROCEDURE   Anterior Cervical Discectomy or Vertebrectomy

Objectives
1. To remove cervical disc or osteophyte causing spinal cord compression, myelopathy, paraparesis, or lateral compression of spinal roots producing pain and weakness in the upper extremity.
2. To remove one or more malignant vertebral bodies.

Position   Supine with head straight forward or slightly turned to the contralateral side. Fix head in a halo or keep in position with skeletal traction, especially if there is fracture dislocation. Provide stockings for intermittent compression of legs during surgery to prevent deep vein thrombosis.

Exposure   The skin of the neck on the operative side.

Incision   Usually a 4–5 cm incision along the skin crease in the proper area for a single-level removal, or a vertical incision along the sternocleidomastoid for a more complicated removal. Hip on one side may also be prepared and draped for removal of bone for grafting, or the lower extremity on one side for the removal of fibular graft.

Preoperative Studies HCT, coagulation profile, electrolytes, BUN, and creatinine plus any other tests indicated by patient's preoperative status.

Blood Bank Order T&C 2 units PRBCs.

Estimated Blood Loss Negligible, unless major vessel is entered or hip graft site is extensive and bleeding occurs from gluteal arteries.

Anesthetic Choice General.

Invasive Monitoring Not necessary.

Airway Considerations The airway is a major consideration here because of problems with mobility of the neck. Need to carefully access airway, range of movement of neck, and symptoms from neck movement. Furthermore, intubation is difficult if head is fixed in a halo before induction. If there is any suspicion of a difficult airway, spontaneous ventilation is the sine qua non for the intubation technique. Fiberoptic bronchoscopic endotracheal intubation may be the optimal approach.

Aspiration Precautions If difficult airway is anticipated, premedicate patient with H_2 receptor blockers or metoclopramide, or both. Use caution in administering premedications that cause respiratory depression in a difficult airway.

Queries for Surgeon Necessary to stabilize neck before induction?

Estimated Surgical Time 3 to 5 hours.

➤ **Anesthetic Considerations**
1. **Anesthetic Concerns**
   a. Airway management, especially as it impacts on already compromised cervical spine.
   b. Dislocation of the spine causing cord compression during intubation or during operation. Movement or coughing during the operation may cause subluxation or dislocation.
   c. Lack of access to head, neck, and airway during procedure.
   d. Arrhythmias and bradycardias elicited by vagal or carotid sinus stimulation in neck.
2. **Anesthetic Technique**
   a. For intubation with spontaneous respiration, ensure a well-anesthetized airway, i.e., topical anesthesia and superior laryngeal nerve and transtracheal block.
   b. Ensure ability for rapid induction (e.g., IV thiopental) immediately after successful intubation to prevent neck movement.
   c. No neck lines on same side as the procedure.
   d. Esophageal stethoscope or nasogastric tube is useful to the surgeon for palpation of esophagus during the neck dissection.
   e. Maintain paralysis intraoperatively.

f. Can use somatosensory evoked potentials (SSEPs) to monitor spinal cord function and integrity. If SSEPs are employed, maintenance of a constant anesthesia level is important.
g. Extubation is a careful, deliberate, planned process because of the difficult airway status.

Intraoperative Hazards

1. Endotracheal tube displacement or disconnection by surgical manipulations around face and neck. Management of an accidental intraoperative extubation takes into consideration the instability of the neck at that moment. Thus, mask ventilation followed by fiberoptic intubation or cricothyrotomy may be the safest approach.
2. Pneumothorax.
3. Injury to neural or vascular structures in neck, namely, injury to recurrent laryngeal nerve (RLN) (causes persistent postextubation hoarseness), unilateral injury to phrenic nerve (generally inconsequential unless patient has poor baseline respiratory function), or injury to major vascular structures (may result in major blood loss).

Postoperative Problems

1. Neurologic deficit
2. Respiratory distress due to
    a. Upper airway compromise, e.g., neck hematoma, bilateral RLN injury
    b. Pulmonary problem, e.g., phrenic nerve injury or pneumothorax

---

SURGICAL PROCEDURE Arteriovenous Malformation (AVM), Craniotomy

---

1. AVMs are congenital vascular lesions providing direct communication between small arteries and veins without intervening capillaries.
2. AVMs could be a single or a multiple unit, vary greatly in size, and may be located anywhere within the cranium.
3. Most common presentation is hemorrhage, either intracerebral or subarachnoid.

Objective   Excision of AVM fistula or elimination of feeding arteries to malformation.

Position   Dependent on location.

Exposure   Dependent on size and location.

Incision   Large scalp flap.

Preoperative Studies   HCT, CXR, ECG, electrolytes, BUN, creatinine.

Blood Bank Order   T&C 4 units PRBCs to be kept available in OR.

Preoperative Medication   Individualize to avoid oversedation.

Estimated Blood Loss Often large and can be massive.

Anesthetic Choice General.

Invasive Monitoring Arterial line and Foley; central venous catheter (CVC). CVC may be helpful in fluid and intravascular volume management.

Airway Considerations Oral endotracheal tube (OETT).

Aspiration Precautions Not necessary unless an emergency procedure or patient is at risk of gastric reflux.

➤ **Anesthetic Considerations**
1. See Aneurysm (Craniotomy).
2. *Risk of rebleeding* in AVM is not as great as in aneurysms.
3. *Prophylactic and therapeutic measures* for risk of excessive bleeding: large-bore IV access, availability of sufficient blood, preoperative collection of autologous units, intraoperative scavenging of blood, and controlled hypotension.
4. *Maintenance* of intracranial hemodynamic stability during induction with special attention to hemodynamics, ventilation, and intracranial pressure (ICP).
5. *Moderate hyperventilation* before surgical dissection aids in surgical exposure.
6. *Hyperperfusion.* Unique to AVM resection is creation of hyperperfusion of normal brain in the area surrounding the resected AVM (reverse steal-type syndrome). Because this results in cerebral edema, avoid postoperative hypertension.

Postoperative Management ICU.

SURGICAL PROCEDURE Brain Biopsy (Open)

To obtain tissue for diagnosis when a neoplasm, infection, or an epileptic focus is suspected.

Position Depends on site of biopsy.

Exposure Area of skull at the site of the disease.

Incision Usually a short incision for burr hole or a skin flap.

Preoperative Studies HCT; coagulation profile optional.

Blood Bank Order T & S or none.

Estimated Blood Loss Negligible.

Anesthetic Choices General or local. Local anesthesia requires good patient access, lighting, and air space. The face contralateral to the site of the lesion is turned to the anesthetist. Monitored anesthesia care is a satisfactory anesthetic for most patients who can cooperate. Sedation should be carefully titrated; access to airway is problematic, especially if stereotactic head frame is placed.

Invasive Monitoring   Not necessary.

Airway Considerations   Oral endotracheal tube (OETT) or monitored anesthesia care.

Aspiration Precautions   Not necessary unless an emergency procedure or the patient is at risk of gastric reflux.

Estimated Surgical Time   Less than 1 hour.

➤ **Anesthetic Considerations**
   1. **Anesthetic Concerns**
      a. ICP considerations may apply.
      b. BP control to decrease risk of bleeding from biopsy site.
      c. Short procedure.
   2. **Anesthetic Technique**
      a. *General:* Smooth induction and emergence in neuroanesthetic fashion. Anesthesia needs to be tailored to awaken patient for neurologic examination at end of procedure.
      b. *Local (monitored care):*
         (1) Administer sedation judiciously: benzodiazepines in an elderly patient may create agitation, whereas oversedation may result in respiratory depression and depressed gag reflexes.
         (2) Take steps to ensure that patient is cooperative.
         (3) Reduce anxiety.
         (4) Establish good air space around face.
         (5) Illuminate area in front of the patient and maintain constant vocal communication as well.

Intraoperative Hazards
   1. Hemorrhage at biopsy site
   2. Patient movement

Postoperative Pain Intensity   Minimal.

Postoperative Pain Control   Routine: codeine 15–30 mg PO or IM q4h often used by neurosurgery services.

SURGICAL PROCEDURE Burr Holes, Trephination, and Craniectomy for Subdural or Epidural Hematoma

Epidural bleeding is almost always from middle meningeal artery. There is an associated fracture across the middle meningeal artery in 75–90% of epidural hematoma cases. Classic picture is loss of consciousness following trauma, then a lucid interval, followed by rapidly progressive neurologic deterioration.

Subdural hematoma may be acute or chronic. Bleeding is from veins between cerebral cortex and dural venous sinuses. Subdural hematomas can follow a trivial and forgotten trauma. Chronic subdural hematomas typically occur in elderly patients. Clinical presentation varies widely, classically with fluctuating signs and symptoms.

Objective To remove spontaneous hematoma or hematoma following trauma.

Position Supine; occasionally lateral or prone, depending on the position of the hematoma.

Exposure One or several burr holes or trephination over the suspected area. In emergency room setting, classic scenario is rapid neurologic deterioration with unilateral pupillary dilatation. A burr hole is made over ipsilateral temporal region.

Blood Bank Order T&S for burr holes. T&C 2 units for craniotomy for hematoma.

Estimated Blood Loss Negligible unless a major sinus has been torn.

Preoperative Studies In emergency setting, none.

Anesthetic Choices General with oral endotracheal intubation. Local anesthesia is practical in an emergency room situation.

Invasive Monitoring Arterial line useful for control of cerebral hemodynamics.

Airway Considerations Associated head and neck injuries. Therefore, rule out neck injury before manipulation of airway.

Aspiration Precautions Full stomach is a consideration because of emergency status and altered mental status. In full stomach and normal airway situations, use modified rapid-sequence induction.

Estimated Surgical Time Less than 1 hour.

➤ **Anesthetic Considerations**
1. **Anesthetic Concerns**
   a. Associated injuries and medical conditions.
   b. Airway and cervical spine considerations.

    c. Intracranial pressure (ICP) control measures: adequate oxygenation, hyperventilation, control of BP, osmotic and loop diuretics, adequate anesthesia. Glucocorticoids are probably not helpful in hematoma- or trauma-related increases in ICP.

    d. Avoid spontaneous bleeding during neurosurgical procedures with general anesthesia.

    e. Keep large-bore IV and blood available if significant bleeding (although rare) or associated injuries are suspected.

    f. Patient may be agitated and have significant hypertension under local anesthesia.

    g. Fatal massive hemorrhage possible in acute cases, especially when skull fracture is present across major venous sinus.

2. Anesthetic Technique

    a. Avoid preoperative sedatives if there is any compromise of mental status.

    b. *Induction:* Proceed in careful smooth induction with special attention to airway and hemodynamic control. Choose drugs with these objectives in mind:

       (1) Ability to awaken patient immediately at end of procedure.

       (2) Lack of access to head after induction.

    c. *Maintenance:* Oxygen; N_2O optional; fentanyl, sufentanil, or alfentanil; low-dose potent volatile agents; short-acting relaxant.

    d. *Emergence:* Aim is to perform neurologic examination immediately after surgery.

Intraoperative Hazards

1. Cerebral edema and increased ICP following removal of hematomas

2. Massive bleeding

3. Patient's movement

4. Blood pressure lability

Postoperative Management   ICU.

Postoperative Problems

1. Intracranial bleeding

2. Depressed mental status

Postoperative Pain Intensity   Minimal.

Postoperative Pain Control   Codeine if mental status permits.

Postoperative Tests   CT scan of head if indicated.

SURGICAL PROCEDURE Cerebrospinal Fluid Shunts:
Ventriculoperitoneal, Ventriculopleural, Ventriculoatrial

Ventriculoperitoneal shunts are the most common.

Objectives
1. To relieve communicating or obstructive hydrocephalus
2. To drain cystic lesions causing increase in intracranial pressure (ICP) and neurologic loss

Position Supine with the head turned to the side opposite the brain compartment to be drained.

Exposure Scalp, back of head, neck, and ear; the anterior thorax and the abdomen for peritoneal shunts. Only the neck and head exposed for ventriculoatrial shunts.

Incision An anterior or posterior scalp incision allows introduction of catheter into the lateral ventricle. An incision to enter a cyst or subdural space is placed appropriately. A subgaleal tunnel is created in back of the ear and down the neck. If drainage site is to be peritoneal cavity, tunneling is continued over the anterior thorax on right. An incision is made in the right side of the abdomen to introduce a peritoneal catheter. Occasionally a catheter is introduced into the pleural space, particularly when the peritoneum is an inappropriate site because of infection or adhesions. Sometimes a catheter is introduced into the right auricle of the heart by entering the jugular vein in the right side of the neck and running it into the heart. After a ventricular catheter is attached to a suitable valve and possibly to an antisiphon device, tubing is burrowed in back of the ear and attached to the connectors running into the atrium, pleural cavity, or peritoneal space. Running the catheters generally requires 1 to 2 cm transverse incisions at long distances apart. If both ventricles must be tapped, a second incision is made on the opposite side of the scalp

Preoperative Studies Routine and as indicated. Patients frequently are elderly and have concurrent diseases. Preoperative testing should be guided accordingly. Generally, all have CT scans of the head worth reviewing.

Blood Bank Order T&S.

Estimated Blood Loss Negligible.

Anesthetic Choice General with oral endotracheal intubation.

Invasive Monitoring None usually.

Airway Considerations Routine.

Aspiration Precautions Depend on neurologic status and urgency of procedure. Patients with high intracranial pressure (ICP) may have symptoms of nausea and vomiting that necessitate rapid sequence induction.

➤ **Anesthetic Considerations**
1. Monitoring intracranial hemodynamics with aim of preventing increases in ICP, especially during smooth induction and emergence.
2. Paralysis and neuromuscular monitoring to avoid patient movement.
3. Short procedure: Aim to avoid long-acting anesthetics and to awaken patient at end of procedure.

Intraoperative Hazards
1. Pneumothorax with ventriculopleural shunts.
2. Venous air embolism with ventriculoatrial shunts.
3. Further increases in ICP during anesthetic.
4. Movement.

Postoperative Problems
1. Intracranial bleeding.
2. Shunt malfunction.

Postoperative Pain Intensity Minimal.

Postoperative Pain Control Often none; codeine.

SURGICAL PROCEDURE Cervical Laminectomy or Foraminotomy, Posterior Approach

After the resection, if instability is present, bony fusion may be carried out. Fusions can be accomplished with iliac crest bone, fibular bone, rib, or methacrylate with wire reinforcement. If posterior fusion is the primary operation, the bones are usually wired to the lamina after the cortices are removed.

Objectives
1. Relief of spinal cord compression and spinal nerve root compression causing pain or neurologic loss.
2. Removal of spinal cord tumors

Position Prone or sitting. If the patient is in the *prone position,* fix the head with a three-point headrest or a horseshoe cerebellar headrest. Elevate chest on rolls or a frame to allow good ventilation and clearance of the head from the operating table. The anesthesiologist may work either at the top of the head while the surgeon works from side to side or at one or the other side of the table while the surgeon works at the head. Occasionally, patients require a halo, head frame, or skeletal traction during the entire procedure. With the prone position and the three-point headrest, ensure that the chin is not hitting the table and that there is good access to the endotracheal tube, which should be suspended on the three-point headrest. Arms usually are by the side, and elbows are not compressed by metal constraints. Depress the shoulders with long adhesive tape running to the base of the table or the footrest. Use intermittent compression stockings during the procedure.
Sitting position offers advantages: Surgeon can operate comfortably. Operative bleeding is minimal, and exposure is optimal because blood drains away from the incision.

Exposure   Back of the shaved head and the neck and upper dorsal thorax. May need iliac, fibular, or rib bone graft.

Incision   Vertical midline incision to expose and remove lamina joints and ligaments and to expose the spinal dura and its roots. High-speed drills are usually used for the bony removal. Soft discs are removed with rongeurs; osteophytes with a high-speed drill, rongeurs, or chisels; and tumors with the classic instruments, ultrasonic aspirators, or laser.

Blood Bank Order   T&C 2 units PRBCs.

Estimated Blood Loss   Less than 500 ml.

Preoperative Studies   HCT, coagulation profile, electrolytes, BUN, creatinine, CXR, neck films.

Anesthetic Choice   General.

Invasive Monitoring   Foley drainage for long procedures and as indicated by position:
1. *Prone position:* Arterial line may be useful but is not necessary.
2. *Sitting position:* Venous air embolus considerations include arterial line, multiorificed central venous catheter (CVC), and precordial Doppler and $ETCO_2$ monitors. Arterial line transducer is placed at level of external meatus of ear.

Airway Considerations   If the patient has a myelopathy or subluxation, awake fiberoptic intubation may be helpful.

Aspiration Precautions   Routine; however, in asleep but spontaneously breathing intubations, H_2 receptor blockers and metoclopramide may be useful.

Queries for Surgeon   Need to stabilize neck?

Estimated Surgical Time   3 to 4 hours average.

➤ **Anesthetic Considerations**
   1. Anesthetic Concerns
      a. Airway management, especially as it impacts on already compromised cervical spine.
      b. Dislocation of the spine that will cause cord compression during intubation or the operation.
      c. Movement or coughing during the operation may cause subluxation or dislocation.
      d. Lack of access to head, neck, and airway during procedure.
      e. Positioning patient—sitting or prone—is difficult, especially in a patient with a compressed cervical spine. Requires additional help and logistics. Pay special attention to pressure points and adequacy of abdominal excursions.
      f. Blood loss increases with unduly high blood pressures.

g. Use of PEEP for patient in sitting position is controversial at best and probably is not recommended. PEEP may increase risk of paradoxical air embolus.

h. Somatosensory evoked potentials (SSEPs) may be used to monitor posterior column function of the spinal cord, thus requiring that a constant level of anesthesia and a low concentration of inhalation agent (<0.75–1.0 minimum alveolar concentration [MAC]) be maintained.

2. **Preoperative Considerations**
Routine history, physical examination, and laboratory studies. Pay special attention to airway examination and associated medical problems. Discuss with patient prospect of awake intubation.

3. **Anesthetic Technique**
a. With spontaneous breathing intubation, ensure good topical anesthesia of airway and ability to rapidly induce general anesthesia after successful endotracheal intubation to prevent neck movement.
b. Positioning is major consideration (pressure points; adequacy of diaphragmatic movement).
c. Intraoperative paralysis is required.
d. If SSEPs are employed, maintain constant anesthesia level.
e. Prevent agitation on emergence.
f. Permit emergence and extubation in supine position, as opposed to prone.
g. Postoperative extubation needs to be careful and deliberate, i.e., performed only in an awake patient.

Intraoperative Hazards
1. Difficult intubation or cervical spine injury with intubation.
2. ETT displacements and disconnections possible with surgical manipulations around face and neck. Accidental intraoperative extubation is a serious problem. With acrobatic skills, reintubation in prone patient may be attempted. Otherwise, turn patient supine immediately, mask ventilate, and, while surgeon is providing neck stabilization, intubate, preferably by fiberoptics, to avoid neck movement. If unable to mask ventilate, cricothyrotomy is necessary.
3. Movement or agitation may result in neck subluxation or dislocation.
4. Neurologic deficit:
   a. Brachial plexus injury
   b. Lateral femoral cutaneous nerve injury
   c. Cervical cord ischemia
5. Pressure point necrosis (chin, face, extremities).
6. *Sitting position—related hazards:*
   a. Venous air embolism
   b. Orthostatic and postinduction hypotension
7. Injury to major vascular structures: rapid blood loss.

Postoperative Pain Intensity   Mild to moderate.

Postoperative Pain Control   Routine.

SURGICAL PROCEDURE Epidural or Subdural Hematoma, Craniotomy

To drain or remove hematoma.

Position Dependent on location of lesion.

Exposure For small hematomas the surrounding area is exposed; for large hematomas the entire side of the head may be draped into the field.

Incision A large craniotomy is used to encompass the abnormal area. Occasionally, burr holes only will be placed if drainage of liquid hematoma is the only goal.

Preoperative Studies HCT, coagulation profile, electrolytes, BUN, creatinine, ECG, CXR. If traumatic injury caused the hematoma, workup is dependent on associated injuries.

Blood Bank Order T&C 2 units PRBCs.

Estimated Blood Loss Minimal to massive. In the usual case, blood loss is negligible. Massive venous hemorrhage occurs when there are skull fractures across the major venous sinuses.

Anesthetic Choice General with oral endotracheal intubation (OETI).

Invasive Monitoring Arterial line and Foley recommended.

Airway Considerations In acute injuries, integrity of cervical spine.

Aspiration Precautions Not necessary unless an emergency procedure or patient is at risk of gastric reflux.

Estimated Surgical Time 1 to 2 hours.

➤ **Anesthetic Considerations**
  1. **Anesthetic Concerns**
     a. Associated injuries (cervical spine and other injuries) or medical conditions (e.g., Stokes Adams syncope as cause of subdural)
     b. Intracranial hemodynamics (i.e., increased intracranial pressure [ICP])
     c. Potential blood loss
     d. Development of cerebral edema immediately following evacuation of hematoma (thus avoid overhydration and hypotonic IV fluids)
  2. **Anesthetic Goals**
     a. In preoperative assessment pay special attention to CNS and cardiovascular status and associated injuries.
     b. Smooth induction and emergence.
     c. Control of hemodynamics (hence, rationale for arterial line for beat-to-beat BP assessment).
     d. Rapid awakening at end of procedure to assess neurologic status.

Intraoperative Hazards
1. Loss of control of airway on induction (dangers of increased Pco_2 and

hypoxemia are compounded in a compromised brain).
2. Loss of hemodynamic control.
3. Sudden blood loss.
4. Air embolism from open venous sinuses.
5. BP drop often follows evacuation of hematoma.

Postoperative Management   ICU. Selected cases may go to less concentrated care areas, especially if subdural hematoma has been chronic.

Postoperative Problems   Hypertension, altered mental status, and decreased airway protection, especially if patient has suffered acute brain injury.

Postoperative Pain Control   Depends on postoperative mental status and airway. Small doses of parenteral narcotics (e.g., codeine) if necessary.

SURGICAL PROCEDURE   Intracranial Pressure Monitoring Device
Placement

Measure intracranial pressure (ICP) by a transcutaneous epidural, subdural, intraparenchymal, or intraventricular catheter measuring device.

Position   Supine.

Exposure   Shaved forehead usually exposed.

Incision   A short incision and a twist drill hole or burr hole are made to allow introduction of the device.

Preoperative Studies   Depend on patient's underlying disease or injuries.

Blood Bank Order   None.

Estimated Blood Loss   Negligible.

Anesthetic Choice   Local; monitored anesthesia care often performed at bedside in ICU.

Invasive Monitoring   Arterial line, Foley, and central venous catheter (CVC). Arterial line BP monitoring will assist in control of ICP by monitoring efficacy of therapy. Such therapy frequently promotes diuresis, making a Foley necessary. A CVC may be helpful to manage volume status.

Airway Considerations   Some of these patients may have head and neck injuries, making airway management difficult. Frequently patients have been intubated already because of altered mental status, need for airway protection, and hyperventilation.

Aspiration Precautions   Often full stomach status.

Estimated Surgical Time   Less than 30 minutes.

➤ **Anesthetic Considerations**
1. Control patient movement and agitation.
2. Control systemic and intracranial hemodynamics.
3. Beware of associated injuries and medical problems.

Intraoperative Hazards
1. Excessive or violent patient movement
2. Detrimental BP and ICP elevations
3. Intracranial bleeding caused by procedure with consequent neurologic deterioration

Postoperative Management   ICU. When ICP needs to be monitored, the patient is usually sick enough to need ICU care. ICP management as necessary with head-up position, hemodynamic optimization, hyperventilation, diuresis, and, in tumor-associated increased ICP, steroids.

Postoperative Problems
1. Dislodgement of arterial line and ICP monitoring due to patient's agitated movements.
2. Associated injuries and medical problems.
3. ICP monitoring device–related infection (meningitis).

Postoperative Pain Intensity   Minor procedure with minimal pain; generally patients are already obtunded.

Postoperative Pain Control   Routine. Patients with elevated ICP may be sensitive to narcotics with respect to depression of respiratory drive.

SURGICAL PROCEDURE   Neoplasms, Craniotomy

Partial or total removal of brain tumors (supratentorial); cure is the objective of total removal.

Position   Depends on the location of the tumor. Head in a three-point headrest. Supine. Table usually flexed. When the body is slightly elevated on one side, a rolled towel is placed just below the axilla that is down to prevent compression of the brachial plexus. Anesthetist is on the side away from the lesion to allow better access to the airway. Provide intermittent compression stockings during surgery and for 12 hours afterward.

Exposure   The midline of the scalp and other key features are marked to exclude all skin but the incisional area.

Incision   Either a straight line, curved, or curvilinear incision is centered over the operative site.

Preoperative Studies   HCT, coagulation profile, glucose, electrolytes, BUN, creatinine, ECG.

Preoperative Medication   Individualized, although patients with intracranial pathology often are sensitive to narcotics. Avoid oversedation. Most patients do not require any sedation.

Blood Bank Order   T&C 2 units PRBCs.

Estimated Blood Loss   Negligible to moderate (200–800 ml).

Anesthetic Choice   General with oral endotracheal tube (OETT). Avoid ketamine; avoid ethrane with hyperventilation (risk of seizure activity); isoflurane is inhalation agent of choice for neuroanesthesia.

Invasive Monitoring   Arterial line; central venous catheter (CVC) optional; Foley.

Airway Considerations   OETT; good control of airway most important for intracranial pressure (ICP) maintenance.

Queries for Surgeon   Require lumbar catheter for CSF drainage?

➤ Anesthetic Considerations
  1. **Anesthetic Goals**
     a. Preoperative assessment and optimization with special attention to neurologic status, signs and symptoms of increased ICP, and associated medical problems.
     b. The crux of the anesthetic technique is minding ICP perioperatively and taking measures to decrease or prevent increases in ICP.
     c. Maintain and monitor for adequate intraoperative paralysis to prevent movement or coughing, which would be disastrous (i.e., surgical mishap or external herniation of brain).
     d. Plan extubation at end of surgical procedure, unless contraindicated, to permit an awake neurologic assessment.
     e. Surgeons often request intraoperative antibiotics, steroids, phenytoin, and diuretics.
  2. **Monitoring**
     a. Routine monitoring plus $ETCO_2$ for hyperventilation purposes.
     b. Arterial line for tight control of intracranial hemodynamics.
     c. Foley necessary because of length of procedure and diuresis.
     d. CVC is useful for fluid management and extensive diuresis.
  3. **Measures to Control or Decrease ICP**
     a. Provide smooth induction and extubation.
     b. Elevate head.
     c. Ensure oxygenation.
     d. Control BP.
     e. Decrease or maintain low airway pressures.
     f. Induce hyperventilation (PCO_2 25–30 mm Hg).
     g. Avoid use of hypoosmotic fluids (recommend normal saline 0.9% for intraoperative IV fluid maintenance).
     h. Administer osmotic and loop diuretics.
     i. Give steroids.
     j. Drain CSF.

   k. Control ICP with thiopental.
   l. Limit inhalation agent concentration.
   m. Avoid histamine-releasing agents (e.g., morphine and curare) and ketamine.

4. **Anesthetic Technique**
   a. Routine patient identification; monitoring of patient.
   b. Establish good IV access.
   c. Sedation (e.g., fentanyl 100 μg or midazolam HCl [Versed] 1 mg).
   d. Place arterial line before induction.
   e. Preoxygenate; deep smooth induction. Typically, thiopental (4–5 mg/kg), vecuronium (0.1 mg/kg), and fentanyl (5–10 μg/kg), or sufentanyl (1–1.5 μg/kg) are used. Lidocaine IV (1 mg/kg) and esmolol (1–2 mg/kg) are optional.
   f. Patient maintained on 50% N_2O, isoflurane, fentanyl (1–2 μg/kg/h), and vecuronium or pancuronium.
   g. Attempt smooth emergence. Patient may benefit from IV lidocaine (1 mg/kg) or esmolol (1–2 mg/kg).
   h. Plan for immediate postoperative neurologic examination.

Intraoperative Hazards
1. Air embolism, hemodynamic lability
2. Movement, with consequent tear of scalp fixation points
3. Straining, with consequent external herniation of brain
4. Hypovolemia or hypokalemia due to diuretics
5. Hyperglycemia with steroids
6. Side effects from mannitol (e.g., hypotension or hypertension or allergic phenomenon)
7. Intraoperative awareness
8. ETT displacement with little access to head
9. Bleeding

Postoperative Management   ICU.

Postoperative Problems
1. *Airway:* Laryngospasm or aspiration.
2. *Cardiovascular system:* Hemodynamic lability due to intravascular volume disturbances, ongoing stimulation (e.g., intubation), preexisting hypertension, CNS-associated ECG abnormalities.
3. *Central nervous system:* Major neurologic deficit, vasospasm, intracranial bleeding, SIADH, hydrocephalus.

Postoperative Pain Intensity   Mild (headache).

Postoperative Pain Control   Routine parenteral.

SURGICAL PROCEDURE Nerve Entrapment Releases

Includes carpal tunnel release of the median nerve, release of the ulnar nerve entrapped in the ulnar groove, and selected distal entrapments of the foot, ankle, and hand.

Objective   To relieve pain and neurologic loss caused by nerve compression in grooves between bones and ligaments. Most common operation is release of the carpal tunnel in the wrist, where the median nerve burrows into the palm to supply sensation to the hand and innervate muscles of the thumb.

Position   Supine. Prone or semiprone for sural nerve harvest.

Incision   Before incision is made, nerve stimulation identifies nerve and measures latencies across block. Linear incision is made in the proper area; nerve is exposed. Nerve excision may be required when a neuroma is present. Nerve grafts may be taken from the lower extremity to bridge the gap, e.g., from the sural nerve.

Preoperative Studies   Routine.

Blood Bank Order   None.

Estimated Blood Loss   Negligible, especially with tourniquet application.

Anesthetic Choices
1. *Hand and elbow operations:* usually local anesthesia with or without a tourniquet.
2. *Leg operations:* usually general anesthesia. General anesthesia may be by mask, laryngeal mask, or endotracheal intubation.
3. *Regional block* is used occasionally. Regional includes nerve blocks or IV regional.

Airway Considerations   Routine.

Aspiration Precautions   Not necessary unless an emergency procedure or patient is at risk of gastric reflux.

Estimated Surgical Time   Approximately 1 hour.

➤ Anesthetic Considerations
1. Distal extremity cases most often done with local or regional anesthesia.
2. Short procedures. Often performed on outpatient basis.
3. Appropriate and adequate duration of regional block (e.g., axillary block with bupivacaine may not be best choice for a short carpal tunnel release).
4. Tourniquet pain common; BP often rises until release of tourniquet.
5. Take special care with IV regional to prevent local anesthetic toxicity from early tourniquet release (i.e., within 20 minutes of IV local anesthetic administration).

Intraoperative Hazards   Local anesthetic toxicity.

SURGICAL PROCEDURE Posterior Fossa Craniotomy for Neoplasms of Skull Base (Acoustic Neuroma, Meningioma)

To remove tumor and spare cranial nerve function.

Position Lateral, sitting, prone.

Exposure Posterior scalp.

Incision Linear, curvilinear, or horseshoe flap. The abdomen may be prepared and draped also to permit the harvesting of the fat pad graft for remedy of spinal fluid rhinorrhea.

Blood Bank Order T&C 2 units PRBCs.

Estimated Blood Loss Minimal.

Preoperative Studies HCT, coagulation profile, electrolytes, BUN, creatinine, ECG. Further preoperative evaluation may be warranted depending on patient's overall status.

Anesthetic Choice General with oral endotracheal intubation.

Invasive Monitoring Arterial line, Foley.

Airway Considerations Fasten tube securely because of difficulty in reintubating patient undergoing craniotomy (sitting, lateral, or prone).

Aspiration Precautions Brainstem involvement may result in loss of airway protection before intubation.

Queries for Surgeon
1. Position for surgery?
2. Will facial nerve stimulation be required?

Estimated Surgical Time Often longer than 6 hours.

➤ **Anesthetic Considerations**
Same as for Neoplasms (Craniotomy) plus issues germane to surgery in sitting position and to the posterior fossa:
1. **Sitting Position Considerations**
   a. *Advantages:* Major advantages are better exposure for surgeon and less bleeding.
   b. *Disadvantages:* Venous air embolus (VAE), orthostatic hypotension, pneumocephalus, cervical cord injury.
   c. *Monitoring:* VAE are detected by Doppler, decreased $ETCO_2$, and decreased SaO_2. Most sensitive is Doppler, then $ETCO_2$. CVC used is multiorificed. CVC positioning can be done by fluoroscopy, x-ray, pressure waveform identification, or ECG-lead identification. Optimal CVC position is junction of superior vena cava and right atrium. Arterial pressure transducer is located at level of ear. Transesophageal echo-

cardiography (TEE) for detection of VAE optional.
d. Response to detected VAE:
   (1) Tell surgeon to flood field.
   (2) Aspirate from CVC.
   (3) Turn off N_2O to avoid air embolus expansion.
   (4) If indicated, compress neck veins (to increase venous back pressure). In ongoing and in severe VAE (rare), it may be necessary to place patient in head-down or left lateral decubitus position to keep air away from right ventricular outflow tract.
2. **Posterior Fossa Considerations**
   Positioning: The anesthetic conduct will depend on the specific position in which the surgery is performed.

Intraoperative Hazards
1. *Cardiovascular System:* Dysrhythmias, bradycardia, asystole; hypotension and hypertension from brainstem surgical manipulation
2. Hypovolemia
3. Bleeding
4. Complications related to sitting position including orthostatic hypotension, nerve compression, and air embolism
5. Patient movement
6. Brainstem injury

Postoperative Management   ICU.

Postoperative Problems
1. *Surgery-related complications:*
   a. Airway compromise, apneic spells, depressed gag reflex, and BP lability can arise from brainstem injury and swelling.
   b. Intracranial bleeding.
   c. Infarction.
2. *Position-related injuries:*
   a. Sciatic nerve, brachial plexus, or ulnar nerve stretch or compression.
   b. Tongue edema from sitting position.
   c. Pneumocephalus is possible, especially with use of N_2O beyond closure of craniotomy.

Postoperative Pain Intensity   Minimal to moderate; incisional.

Postoperative Pain Control   Routine parenteral.

SURGICAL PROCEDURE Stereotactic Surgery

Stereotactic surgery involves three steps:
1. Placement in head frame with local anesthesia; IV sedation optional.
2. Imaging studies (CT/MRI) done the day before or the day of surgery.
3. Surgical procedure.

Objective   To produce a brain lesion to relieve tremor, rigidity, or other abnormal movements in patients with Parkinson's disease, dystonia, musculorum deformans, or a related condition. Also used to obtain an excisional biopsy specimen of a neoplasm or for resection of a cerebral mass lesion.

Stereotactic surgery allows access to deep structures without damage to surrounding neurologic structure.

Position   Supine. A stereotactic head frame is attached to the skull through the skull fixation points.

Exposure   Entire scalp is available to the surgeon.

Blood Bank Order   T&S.

Estimated Blood Loss   Negligible.

Anesthetic Choices   Local with IV sedation for stereotactic frame placement and imaging technique and for some stereotactic surgery. Most stereotactic surgery is done with patient under general anesthesia. Patients unable to cooperate (children or those with a severe motor disorder) are given general anesthesia for frame placement and imaging.

Invasive Monitoring   Arterial line indicated for surgical procedure when ABGs or beat-to-beat BP measurement is desirable.

Airway Considerations   Airway management is difficult in a patient in a stereotactic head frame. In an emergency situation, airway management may require partial or complete removal of the head frame.

Aspiration Precautions   Routine.

Estimated Surgical Time   Variable.

➤ **Anesthetic Considerations**
Hypertension during insertion of the electrode may cause bleeding along the electrode track. Failure to sedate the patient may lead to dislodgement of the stereotactic device.
1. **Preoperative Assessment**
   Routine history, physical examination, and laboratory studies. Pay particular attention to associated medical problems, neurologic status, and suitability for IV sedation.
2. **Monitoring**
   During IV sedation or general anesthesia, adhere to full routine monitoring (anesthesia personnel present at all times, BP cuff, ECG, pulse oximeter, precordial stethoscope). Additionally, during general anesthesia,

continuously monitor $ETCO_2$ along with ventilation and CO_2 control.

3. **Sedation**

   Local and IV sedation used during head-frame placement, imaging studies, and occasionally during surgical procedure. IV sedation by anesthesiologist typically involves benzodiazepines and barbiturates or narcotics or both. Maintain patient awake, responsive, and sedated except during intensely uncomfortable moments. Ultra-short-acting agent (e.g., propofol or barbiturates) may be especially useful.

4. **General Anesthesia**

   General anesthesia with oroendotracheal intubation required for most of the actual stereotactic surgical procedure, except thalamotomies and shunt placement which are performed under local and IV sedation. If head frame is off, general anesthesia is induced before head-frame placement. If head frame is in place, range of neck motion and access to mouth are extremely limited, even with the anterior piece off. These patients are fiberoptically intubated while spontaneous ventilation is maintained.

5. **Emergence**

   The goal is for immediate postoperative awakening for brief neurologic examination.

Intraoperative Hazards

1. Panic reaction
2. Claustrophobia at any time
3. Loss of consciousness or airway or inadequate gas exchange requiring emergency intubation
4. Intracranial hemorrhage—most frequent complication—accounts for most morbidity and mortality
5. Other complications: seizures, neurologic deficits, skull perforation from pins

Postoperative Management   ICU.

Postoperative Problems   Venous air embolism from pinholes after frame is removed.

Postoperative Pain Intensity   None to minimal.

SURGICAL PROCEDURE Thoracic Disc Disease: Thoracotomy or Retroperitoneal Approach

Indicated for lumbar fusion, thoracic disc tumors, or other thoracic spine disease (e.g., tuberculosis).

Objectives
1. To remove a disc protrusion pressing against the thoracic or high lumbar spinal canal that can or actually is causing paraparesis
2. To remove a diseased vertebral body
3. To create an anterior spinal fusion

Anterolateral approaches also are used to expose infections such as tuberculosis and occasionally are used to fuse lumbar spinal vertebral bodies in patients with unstable backs from disc disease. *Rationale:* To gain access to the ventral spinal canal, where the actual compression is taking place, rather than attacking the ventral process from the posterior approach, as in laminectomy. Surgeon gets better view of the affected area, which prevents damage to the spinal cord.

Position The patient generally is placed in an oblique anterolateral position with the chest elevated partially or fully by rolls placed against the back. Patient thus may be fully lateral or semisupine to give the surgeon access to the rib cage and to permit an incision from 4 to 5 cm lateral to the midline of the back and then obliquely forward along the ribline to the sternum.

Exposure Iliac spine to axilla and contralateral nipple to scapula or posterior midline.

Incision Thoracotomy for removal of rib back to the vertebral body. High speed drills are used to remove portions of the vertebral body to expose the ventral surfaces of the spinal canal where the spinal dura is found. Soft disc or vertebral body is removed. More extensive surgery may be required in cases of tuberculosis or osteomyelitis. Requirement for bony fusion depends on the amount of vertebral body removed; bone generally is taken from ipsilateral iliac crest. Wound is closed, and a pleural vacuum tube is left in place to ensure full inflation of the lung. During the operation the ipsilateral lung is partially collapsed.

Preoperative Studies CBC, electrolytes, glucose, BUN, creatinine, CXR, ECG; PFTs and ABGs if indicated. Workup may include CT scan and MRI, as well as a metastatic workup.

Blood Bank Order T&C 3 units PRBCs; keep 3 units PRBCs in reserve in case needed.

Estimated Blood Loss Minimal, unless a major vessel is entered.

Anesthetic Choices General only; or combined regional and general.

Invasive Monitoring Arterial line; Foley if protracted procedure.

Airway Considerations   Oral endotracheal tube (OETT); single-lung ventilation.

Aspiration Precautions   Not necessary unless an emergency procedure or patient is at risk of gastric reflux.

Queries for Surgeon   Need for DLETT to facilitate exposure?

Estimated Surgical Time   4 to 6 hours.

➤ **Anesthetic Considerations**
1. **Preoperative Considerations**
   Accurate delineation of preoperative neurologic deficit and associated medical problems.
2. **Intraoperative Considerations**
   a. See General Considerations, Chapter 3, Thoracic Procedures.
   b. Anterolateral positioning: pressure point protection, nerve injury protection, and respiratory compromise.
   c. Single-lung ventilation may be required.
   d. Paralysis is recommended for surgical exposure, prevention of sudden patient movement or gasp with possible entrainment of venous air embolism.
   e. Early awakening after surgery for neurologic examination.
   f. Somatosensory evoked potentials (SSEPs) may be required or useful. SSEPs consist of stimulation of major peripheral nerves with subcortical potentials (head, neck, and spine) and cortical potentials (scalps) recorded. Chief factors affecting SSEPs are inhalation anesthetics, barbiturates, benzodiazepines, and temperature changes. Most importantly, SSEPs require constant level of anesthesia and less than 0.75–1.0 minimum alveolar concentration (MAC) of inhalation anesthesia.
   g. Immediate postoperative neurologic evaluation, especially of lower extremities, requires anesthetic technique with rapid postoperative awakening.

Intraoperative Hazards
1. Desaturation caused by double-lumen endotracheal tube (DLETT) displacement. Intraoperative DLETT desaturation management:
   a. Ensure 100% F_{IO_2}.
   b. Check proper ETT placement.
   c. Suction secretions.
   d. Up-lung CPAP.
   e. Down-lung PEEP.
   f. Intermittent breath to up lung.
2. Patient movement with risk of surgical mishap.

Postoperative Management   ICU.

Postoperative Pain Intensity   Severe.

Postoperative Pain Control   Routine: PCA; intercostal nerve blocks; intrapleural catheter; epidural catheter.

Postoperative Tests   CXR, HCT, ABGs.

SURGICAL PROCEDURE   Transsphenoidal Tumor Resection

Objectives
1. Total or subtotal removal of intrasellar or suprasellar tumor, pituitary adenomas or craniopharyngioma
2. Drainage of cyst

Position   Supine: head elevated and straight or turned to the side of the surgeon. Secure endotracheal tube on side opposite to the surgeon. Image amplifier usually placed in the lateral position opposite to patient's head. The anesthetist in most cases is to left side of patient. Can be exposed to radiographic beam unless protected by apron or lead stand.

Exposure   Patient's face, nose, and mouth are exposed. The lower right quadrant of the abdomen is usually draped in to allow the harvesting of a fat pad graft.

Incision   Cocaine packing or epinephrine infiltration of the mucosa of the gingiva or nasal mucosa is used. Incision is made either in the left nostril or the midline septum of the nose, or if the oral approach is used, along the gingiva above the upper incisors. An abdominal incision to remove fat pad graft is usually made in the right lower quadrant or right thigh.

Preoperative Studies   HCT, platelets, PTT, PT, electrolytes, BUN, creatinine, glucose. Neurologic workup would include CT scan with contrast or MRI, or both.

Blood Bank Order   T&C 2 units PRBCs.

Estimated Blood Loss   Negligible, unless major vessel is injured.

Anesthetic Choice   General anesthesia with oral endotracheal intubation (OETT).

Invasive Monitoring   None necessary; arterial line optional.

Airway Considerations   Oral endotracheal tube (OETT). Necessitates oral intubation; preformed or reinforced endotracheal tube (ETT) useful. Airway considerations for acromegaly are macroglossia, prognathism, pharyngeal and epiglottic soft tissue hypertrophy, and laryngeal stenosis.

Aspiration Precautions   Not necessary unless an emergency procedure or patient is at risk of gastric reflux.

Queries for Surgeon Use of visual evoked potentials? (Rarely used because difficult to interpret).

Estimated Surgical Time Variable, 3 to 4 hours.

➤ **Anesthetic Considerations**
1. **Preoperative Evaluation**
   Associated medical conditions: steroid dependence; syndrome of inappropriate antidiuretic hormone (SIADH) with resultant hyponatremia and hypokalemia; hypopituitarism with resultant Addison's disease and diabetes insipidus; acromegaly with eosinophilic adenoma and consequent airway considerations; other hormone-producing tumors such as Cushing's (ACTH) or prolactinomas. Pituitary tumors rarely associated with increased intracranial pressure (ICP).
2. **Anesthetic Problems**
   a. Airway and ETT considerations mentioned above.
   b. ICP precautions in patients suspected of increased ICP (i.e., close BP control, diuretics, head elevation, hyperventilation, deep induction, limited use of inhalation agents).
   c. Sitting or head-up position considerations (i.e., nerve compression, postural hypotension, and venous air embolism).
   d. Migration of tip of ETT with head movement (downward ETT movement with flexion and upward ETT movement with extensor; 0 to 4 cm excursion).
   e. Lack of access to head and neck during surgical procedure.
   f. No nasal instruments (e.g., temperature probe).
   g. Surgeon's use of submucosal epinephrine or cocaine may sensitize myocardium to arrhythmias (especially with halothane).
   h. Blood in stomach induces nausea and vomiting.
   i. Patient should be awake and alert at end of procedure. Postextubation breathing difficulty may be due to failure to remove pharyngeal pack or to laryngospasm from blood or other foreign body in pharynx.
3. **Anesthetic Technique**
   In patients with pituitary tumor who are otherwise healthy, use general anesthesia with OETT and pharyngeal pack placement. Specific monitoring for venous air embolism (Doppler, arterial line, $ETCO_2$) generally not required. Low risk of venous air embolism even in head-up position. Muscle paralysis and neuromuscular monitoring recommended to prevent sudden patient movement. Ensure removal of pharyngeal packs before extubation. Ensure anesthetic technique that allows rapid awakening to permit neurologic examination immediately after surgery.

Intraoperative Hazards
1. ETT displacement or disconnection by surgeon.
2. Intracranial bleeding.
3. Patient's moving, which exposes patient to risk of surgical mishap.

Postoperative Problems
1. Development of endocrine problems, such as diabetes insipidus, and Addison's disease.
2. Damage to optic nerve or chiasm.
3. Intracranial bleeding.

4. Persistent CSF leak.
5. Infection.

Postoperative Pain Intensity   Minimal.

Postoperative Pain Control   Parenteral narcotics (e.g., codeine).

SURGICAL PROCEDURE   Trigeminal Thermal Rhizotomy (Patient Sedated)

Surgeon introduces a long needle through the mucosa under the upper lip on the appropriate side, advancing it by radiographic guidance to the foramen ovule. By stimulation and the aspiration of cerebrospinal fluid or by radiographic verification, the proper site for heating the nerve is determined. Procedure generally is done with the patient awake enough to determine by stimulation the proper localization of the electrode. Surgeon sometimes can tell by erythema in the proper facial area such as the cheek, chin, or forehead or by pain stimulation of these areas that the rhizotomy is properly done.

Objective   Partial denervation of trigeminal nerve for tic douloureux by insertion of an electrode into the foramen ovale and induction of radiofrequency heat lesions.

Position   These procedures are generally done in the radiology suite.

Exposure   Midface area.

Preoperative Studies   Depend on patient's preexisting medical problems.

Blood Bank Order   None.

Estimated Blood Loss   Negligible.

Anesthetic Choices   Local anesthesia, with occasional administration of sedation and narcotic agents during periods of intense discomfort. Sedation can consist of ultra-short-acting agent such as barbiturate (thiopental or methohexital) or propofol for periods of intense discomfort

Invasive Monitoring   None.

Airway Considerations   None.

Aspiration Precautions   Patients have an unprotected airway during lesioning episodes, when an ultra-short-acting agent is given. This is not a problem unless the patient is at risk of regurgitation.

Estimated Surgical Time   30 minutes to 1 hour.

▶ **Anesthetic Considerations**
1. IV sedation requires that an anesthesiologist be present.
2. Patient needs to be able to communicate with surgeon during procedure.

Intraoperative Hazards
1. Excessive IV sedation
2. Agitation or anesthetic mishap requiring induction of general anesthesia

Postoperative Management To floor; no need for PACU unless patient is oversedated.

Postoperative Pain Intensity Mild.

SUGGESTED READING
General Review
Shapiro H, Drummond JC. Neurosurgical Anesthesia and Intracranial Hypertension. In Miller RD (ed). New York: Churchill Livingstone, 1990.

Aneurysm (Craniotomy), Arteriovenous Malformation
Black S. Cerebral Aneurysm and Arteriovenous Malformation. In Cucchiara R, Michenfelder JD (eds), Clinical Neuroanesthesia. New York: Churchill Livingstone, 1990.
Wilkins RH. Natural History of Intracranial Vascular Malformation: A Review. Neurosurgery 16:421, 1985.
Willatts S, Walters F. Anesthesia for Vascular Surgery. In Willatts S, Walters F (eds), Anesthesia and Intensive Care for the Neurosurgical Patient. Oxford: Blackwell Scientific Publications, 1986.

Anterior Cervical Discectomy, Cervical Laminectomy (Posterior Approach), Thoracic Disc Disease
Cucchirara RF. Safety of the Sitting Position. Anesthesiology 61:790, 1984.
Horlocker T, Cucchiara RF, Ebersold M. Vertebral Column and Spinal Cord Surgery. In Cucchiara RF, Michenfelder JD (eds), Clinical Neuroanesthesia. New York: Churchill Livingstone, 1990.
Willatts S, Walters F. Anesthesia for Spinal Surgery. In Willatts S, Walters F (eds), Anesthesia and Intensive Care for the Neurosurgical Patient. Oxford: Blackwell Scientific Publications, 1986.

Intracranial Pressure Monitoring Device Placement
Sullivan HG, Motte PS, Allison JD, Becker DF. Intracranial Pressure Monitoring and Interpretation. In Cottrell JD, Turndorf H (eds), Anesthesia and Neurosurgery. St Louis: CV Mosby, 1986.

Neoplasms (Craniotomy), Brain Biopsy
Black S, Cucchiara RF. Tumor Surgery. In Cucchiara RF, Michenfelder JD, Clinical Neuroanesthesia. New York: Churchill Livingstone, 1990.
Michenfelder JD. Anesthesia and the Brain. New York: Churchill Livingstone, 1988.

Posterior Fossa (Craniotomy)

Campkin TV. The Sitting Position. In Anderton JM, Keen RI, Neave R (eds), Positioning the Surgical Patient. London: Butterworths, 1988.

Matjasko J, Petrozza P, Cohen M, Steinberg P. Anesthesia and Surgery in the Seated Position: Analysis of 554 Cases. Neurosurgery 17:695, 1985.

Stereotactic Surgery

Manniner P, Contreras J. Anesthetic Considerations for Craniotomy in Awake Patients. Int Anesthesiol Clin 24:157, 1986.

Perkins W, Kelly P, Faust RJ. Stereotactic Surgery. In Cucchiara RF, Michenfelder JD (ed), Clinical Neuroanesthesia. New York: Churchill Livingstone, 1990.

Transphenoidal Tumor Resection

Post KD, Newfield P. Transphenoidal Procedures. In Newfield P, Cottrell J (eds), Handbook of Neuroanesthesia: Clinical and Physiologic Principles. Boston: Little, Brown & Co., 1983.

Trigeminal Thermal Rhizotomy

Patt R. Neurosurgical Interventions for Chronic Pain Problems. In Frost F (ed), Anesthesia Clinics of North America. Philadelphia: W.B. Saunders, vol. 5, Sept 1987.

CHAPTER 7

OBSTETRIC AND GYNECOLOGIC PROCEDURES

SURGICAL PROCEDURE Cesarean Section

C-sections account for 10% to 30% of all deliveries in the United States.

Objective   Termination of pregnancy from abdominal approach. Major indications for C-section are dystocias (one third of cases), previous C-section (one fourth of cases), fetal distress, and breech presentation. Other indications are prolapsed cord, placenta previa, and genital herpes.

Position   Lateral uterine displacement.

Exposure   Pubic area to xiphoid.

Incision
1. Low transverse incision for low cervical approach is most common.
2. Vertical incision for rapid entry is classic approach.

Blood Bank Order   T&S.

Estimated Blood Loss   500 to 1000 ml.

Preoperative Studies   HCT, coagulation profile, electrolytes, BUN, creatinine, glucose, FHR strip or auscultation records. There may be no time for preoperative studies for STAT C-sections.

Anesthetic Choices   Regional, general, or local.
1. Regional (most common): spinal or epidural block. *Epidural level* T4 to T6 block for surgery requires higher concentration of local anesthetic than for labor analgesia, i.e., 2% with 1:200,000 epinephrine vs 1% lidocaine; or 0.5% vs 0.125% bupivicaine. *Spinal anesthesia* advantages, preferably performed with thin spinal needle, are rapid onset, dense dependable block, little maternal and fetal drug exposure, preservation of airway reflexes, relative simplicity of technique. Regional anesthesia is contraindicated in severe coagulopathy, patient refusal, increased intracranial pressure (ICP) with mass lesion, sepsis or infection at lumbar area, progressive

neurologic disease, hemodynamic instability, severe aortic stenosis, and idiopathic hypertrophic subaortic stenosis (IHSS).
2. General anesthesia (GA) with endotracheal intubation (ETI). GA requires ETI.
3. Local (rare).

Invasive Monitoring   None, unless indicated by associated medical conditions. *Preeclampsia management:* In severe preeclampsia a Foley, central venous catheter (CVC), and arterial line are recommended. If preeclamptic patient develops oliguria, congestive heart failure (CHF), or hemodynamic instability, a pulmonary artery catheter (PAC) is desirable.

Airway Considerations   Because airway of a pregnant patient is complicated by edema of mucosal membranes, a small endotracheal tube (ETT) (6.5–7.0 inner diameter) is required; risk of mucosal bleeding with nasal ETT is greater because mucous membranes are more friable. Weight gain and engorged breasts may render laryngoscopy more difficult.
   Failed intubation protocol: Don't attempt intubation more than twice. Maintain cricoid pressure and attempt mask ventilation. If mask ventilation also is unsuccessful, a surgical airway (e.g., cricothyroid puncture or cricothyrotomy) is required (although may attempt laryngeal airway before surgical airway). On the other hand, if able to mask ventilate and C-section is elective, wake patient and intubate by awake and spontaneous ventilation technique or use regional technique. If able to mask ventilate and C-section is an emergency procedure, maintain cricoid pressure and use mask anesthetic; paralysis optional.

Aspiration Precautions   Full stomach (pulmonary acid aspiration syndrome [Mendelson's syndrome]). All patients pregnant approximately 16 weeks are considered at high risk of aspiration because of lower esophageal sphincter relaxation, increased abdominal pressure, and high incidence of esophageal reflux.

➤ **Anesthetic Considerations**
1. **Preoperative Considerations**
   Routine evaluation plus gestational history and assessment of fetal well-being (fetal movements, ultrasound results, FHR strips). High-risk pregnancy comprises virtually any maternal, uterine, or fetal disorder (e.g., diabetes mellitus, hypertension, placenta previa, small-for-gestational-age fetus).
2. **Anesthetic Concerns**
   a. Maternal
      (1) Gestational physiology.
      (2) Airway.
      (3) *Cardiovascular system:* increased cardiac output, increased blood volume, aortocaval compression syndrome; ephedrine is vasopressor of choice (over pure alpha agonist).
      (4) *Respiratory system:* decreased functional residual capacity, increased $\dot{V}O_2$, hyperventilation (increased minute ventilation).
      (5) *Central nervous system:* increased sensitivity to local anesthetics and decreased minimum alveolar concentration (MAC).
      (6) *Hematologic system:* physiologic anemia and increasing tendency to thrombosis.

(7) *Uterus:* blood flow is not autoregulated and therefore is pressure dependent.
  b. Fetal: All drugs are assumed to pass through the placenta (N.B. neuromuscular blockers pass minimally).
3. **Anesthetic Technique for General Anesthesia (GA)**
  a. Administer nonparticulate antacids, e.g., sodium citrate 30 ml.
  b. Place monitors and establish large-bore IV.
  c. Prehydrate, e.g., with 1 L crystalloid.
  d. Lateral uterine displacement.
  e. Preoxygenate.
  f. Surgeon and nurses scrub and abdomen is prepped and draped before GA induction to keep time from induction to delivery at <8 minutes. More important, time from uterine incision to delivery should be kept at <3 minutes. A prolonged uterine-incision-to-delivery time is associated with fetal acidosis and an Apgar score lower than would otherwise be expected.
  g. *Induction:* Rapid-sequence induction with cricoid pressure, thiopental (average dose 3–4 mg/kg), and succinylcholine (1 mg/kg).
  h. Incision is made after you confirm bilateral breath sounds and release cricoid pressure.
  i. *Maintenance:* Maintain anesthesia with 50% N_2O, 50% oxygen, and 0.75% isoflurane or 1% enflurane until delivery. After delivery, administer oxytocin and narcotics. Nondepolarizing relaxants and antibiotics are administered if requested by surgeon. Maintain normocapnia.
  j. Extubate patient awake only.
4. **Anesthetic Technique for Regional Anesthesia**
  a. Review history, physical examination, and laboratory studies and obtain consent.
  b. *Preinduction:* Administer nonparticulate antacid (sodium citrate 30 ml), place monitors, establish large-bore IV (e.g., 14 or 16 G preferably), prehydrate with 1 L Ringer's lactate, and administer oxygen by mask.
  c. *Induction:* Place epidural or spinal with patient sitting or in lateral decubitus position. *Epidural block:* Establish with 2% lidocaine with 1: 200,000 epinephrine or with 2–3% chloroprocaine to a T4–T6 level. Avoid epinephrine in preeclampsia. *Spinal anesthesia:* Establish with lidocaine 5% in 7.5% dextrose (average dose 75 mg) or with bupivacaine (12–15 mg).
  d. *Maintenance:* Maintain patient in lateral uterine displacement until baby is born. After delivery, obstetrician typically asks for oxytocin (10–20 units in IV bag); antibiotics (e.g., cefoxitin or cefazolin) optional. Once infant is delivered, patient may receive sedative (e.g., droperidol, fentanyl, midazolam) as necessary. Routine fluid requirement is approximately 2–3 L crystalloid.

Intraoperative Hazards
1. Maternal
  a. Failed intubation.
  b. Aspiration on induction or extubation.
  c. Maternal agitation or nausea and vomiting with regional. Suspect hypotension or vagal reaction from peritoneal traction during uterine exteriorization when patient has nausea and vomiting.

d. Significant bleeding.
e. Maternal awareness with GA.
f. Failed regional (too high, too low, patchy, no block at all).
2. Fetal
    a. Fetal head entrapment.
    b. Neonatal resuscitation. Neonate may need resuscitation; call for help and have neonate brought to head of bed near mother. Ask nurse to watch over mother while you resuscitate neonate. Do not abandon unstable mother to resuscitate neonate. Your responsibility is first to the mother and second to the neonate at all times.

Postoperative Pain Intensity   Moderate.

Postoperative Pain Control   Spinal opioids, PCA, or IM narcotics. Patients who have undergone C-sections with regional technique are suitable candidates for postoperative spinal opioids. Low incidence of respiratory depression with epidural narcotic in postpartum period because of progesterone's respiratory stimulant effect.

Postoperative Tests   HCT, glucose, Rh blood type of infant.

SURGICAL PROCEDURE   Dilatation and Curettage (D&C)

Indications
1. Incomplete or therapeutic abortion
2. Postmenopausal bleeding
3. Menorrhagia or metrorrhagia
Therapeutic abortions can be done safely at 8 to 20 weeks' gestation, although restrictions apply at some institutions.

Objective   Evaluation of uterus. Involves evaluating contents and scraping out lining of endometrium. It is routine for the surgeon to perform an examination while patient is under anesthesia and completely relaxed.

Position   Lithotomy.

Exposure   Perineum.

Blood Bank Order   May want to crossmatch several units if patient has been bleeding significantly. Otherwise, T&S.

Estimated Blood Loss   Depends on indication for procedure and weeks of gestation.

Preoperative Studies   HCT, coagulation profile.

Anesthetic Choices
1. *General anesthesia* most often by mask. Endotracheal intubation used for patients at risk for aspiration (e.g., reflux symptoms or if >16 weeks' gestation).
2. *Regional* (e.g., spinal with lidocaine 5%) indicated as an alternative to general anesthesia or local technique.
3. *Local with IV sedation* (e.g., fentanyl 1 μg/kg and midazolam 1–2 mg IV) commonly used at gynecology clinics without anesthesia personnel.

Invasive Monitoring   None.

▶ **Anesthetic Considerations**
1. **Anesthetic Goals**
   a. Alleviate patient anxiety; often one is dealing with a young woman undergoing an emotionally and psychologically taxing situation i.e., therapeutic abortion or D&C for incomplete abortion.
   b. Short procedure (1 to 10 minutes).
   c. Provide analgesia. Amnesia and loss of consciousness for GA.
   d. Facilitate surgical exposure by providing adequate depth of anesthesia. Lightly anesthetized patients adduct legs as surgeon begins cervical dilatation.
2. **Preoperative Evaluation**
   Routine history, physical examination, laboratory studies, and patient consent. Pay special attention to duration and quantity of vaginal bleeding (e.g., number of soaked pads, general appearance, e.g., pale or orthostatic symptoms), history of esophageal reflux or hiatal hernia, vital signs, airway, HCT, coagulation profile, patient's anesthetic preference.
3. **Anesthetic Technique for General Anesthesia**
   a. Routine monitoring and IV access.
   b. IV induction with fentanyl 1 μg/kg and a reduced dose of propofol, e.g., 1 to 2 mg/kg, or other induction agent.
   c. *Maintenance:* N_2O and IV anesthesia (e.g., propofol, alfentanyl) or volatile agent. Deepen anesthesia just before cervical dilatation, which is the greatest stimulus. May use small doses of succinylcholine (10 mg IV) to facilitate mask ventilation and prevent or treat laryngospasm.
   d. Turn off volatile anesthetic in middle of curettage to allow rapid awakening. Too rapid awakening, however, causes patient straining and regurgitation and increases potential for aspiration.

Intraoperative Hazards
1. Bleeding
2. Patient movement
3. Uterine perforation
4. Laryngospasm
5. Vomiting and unprotected airway

SURGICAL PROCEDURE Laparoscopic Surgery

Includes diagnostic laparoscopy, laparoscopic tubal ligation, laparoscopic cholecystectomy, laparoscopic appendectomy, and more laparoscopic procedures to come.

Comments: Laparoscopic techniques are gaining in popularity. *Advantages:* smaller incisions, less postoperative pain, decreased risk of postoperative respiratory compromise, faster recovery, and lower health care costs because of shorter hospital stays. *Disadvantages:* technically more difficult, limited surgical exposure, increased risk of cardiorespiratory compromise, and higher setup costs.

Objectives
1. Exploration for diagnostic evaluation
2. Surgery via laparoscope

Position   Supine or lithotomy with Trendelenburg or reverse Trendelenburg.
1. *Gynecologic laparoscopy:* Trendelenburg (head-down) in supine or lithotomy position because abdominal viscera must remain out of pelvis for surgical exposure. Consider potential for respiratory compromise due to cephalad movement of diaphragm.
2. *General surgery laparoscopy:* Supine, with or without reverse Trendelenburg (head-up), which minimizes respiratory compromise.

Exposure   Periumbilical and area of surgery.

Incision
1. *Gynecologic:* Lower quadrant, midline puncture.
2. *General:* Puncture at or near area of surgery.

Blood Bank Order
Gynecologic and General: T&S.

Estimated Blood Loss   Minimal.

Preoperative Studies   Routine. *Laparoscopic cholecystectomy:* CBC, LFTs, coagulation profile, electrolytes, BUN, creatinine, glucose.

Anesthetic Choices   General or regional. General anesthesia preferred. Regional (epidural) is feasible but requires cooperative and motivated patient who is free of significant respiratory disease. Regional is poorly tolerated because of increased ventilatory load from insufflated CO_2 and Trendelenburg position. Also, patient should be forewarned of respiratory discomfort and possible shoulder pain from referred diaphragmatic irritation.

Invasive Monitoring   Routine monitoring.

Aspiration Precautions   Endotracheal intubation necessary: high intraabdominal pressures increase risk of passive gastroesophageal reflux and impede ventilation.

Estimated Surgical Time
1. Gynecology: 15 to 60 minutes.
2. General: 1 to 4 hours.
   Comments: Preoperative diagnosis and surgeon's skill are best predictors of time required.

➤ **Anesthetic Considerations**
1. **Risks Associated with CO_2 Insufflation**
   a. Respiratory compromise
      (1) Depends on position (worse with Trendelenburg).
      (2) Increased CO_2 load requires larger minute volume.
      (3) Risk of intraoperative pneumothorax, pneumoperitoneum.
   b. CO_2 venous air embolism. CO_2 air embolism can occur through venous sinuses or perforation of a vein resulting in sudden increase in $ETCO_2$ and air embolism syndrome.
   c. Hemodynamic compromise. Intraabdominal pressure (IAP) >30 mm Hg decreases cardiac output and diminishes venous return. Ideal IAP is unknown, although 15 mm Hg is a "safe" figure. Continuously monitor CO_2 insufflation pressure. Tachycardia is common (possibly from surgical stimulation of celiac plexus). On insertion of trochar, vagal reflex initiates bradycardia, leading to asystole. Hypercapnia increases risk of arrhythmias.
2. **Patient Movement**
   Paralysis recommended since sudden patient movement with sharp instruments in abdomen may result in hemorrhage or perforation or electrical burns of a viscus.
3. **$ETCO_2$ Monitoring**
   $ETCO_2$ should be monitored for
   a. Respiratory compromise
   b. Absorption of insufflated CO_2 in abdomen
   c. CO_2 air embolism

Postoperative Problems
1. Nausea and vomiting. Antiemetics may reduce incidence.
2. Shoulder pain. Referred diaphragmatic irritation is best relieved by removing all intraabdominal CO_2 and air before closure of abdomen.
3. Intraabdominal bleeding. Hypotension in postoperative period may be due to intraabdominal hemorrhage.
4. Bile leaks. Acute abdomen or peritonitis may be late signs of bile leaks.
5. Pain control. Often minor pain; treated with nonnarcotics or narcotics.

SURGICAL PROCEDURE Nonobstetric Anesthesia for Pregnant Patient

Comments: 2% of pregnant patients require anesthesia for nonobstetric surgical procedures. No association has been established between anesthesia and premature labor, fetal death, or teratogenicity. Surgical procedures, however, are closely related to premature labor and fetal death. Premature contractions can be terminated with a tocolytic agent (ritodrine or terbutaline). Yet even neurosurgery and cardiac surgery can be performed without harm to fetus.

Objective Most common reasons for surgery are cervical cerclage, trauma, appendicitis, and ovarian cyst.

Position Depends on procedure. After the first trimester the patient should not be positioned supine but rather in the lateral uterine displacement position.

Preoperative Studies Depend on procedure. Minimal laboratory requirements are HCT, coagulation profile, glucose, BUN, creatinine, urinalysis. CXR not recommended.

Blood Bank Order Depends on procedure.

Anesthetic Choices Local, regional, or general. Elective surgery is deferred until after delivery. Nonurgent surgery is deferred until after the critical period of organogenesis (15 to 55 days' gestation). Regional anesthesia (especially spinal) is probably preferable, since it exposes fetus to least amount of drug. No anesthetic drug is contraindicated, but avoid high doses of ketamine (>1 mg/kg), as it may increase uterine tone.

Invasive Monitoring Depends on procedure. Noninvasive intraoperative and postoperative monitoring should include Doppler fetal heart rate (FHR) at ≥16 weeks' gestation, and in third trimester it should include tocodynamometric (i.e., uterine tone) monitoring if possible.

Aspiration Precautions After 16 weeks' gestation.

➤ **Anesthetic Considerations**
  1. **Pregnancy Considerations**
     a. Preoperative nonparticulate antacid requirement.
     b. Edematous airways; therefore use small endotracheal tube (ETT) because of risk of bleeding from edematous mucosa, and avoid nasal endotracheal intubation (ETI).
     c. Supine hypotension syndrome.
     d. Rapid maternal desaturation on induction after 20 weeks' gestation because of decreased functional residual capacity (FRC) and increased oxygen requirement.
     e. Ephedrine is vasopressor of choice.
     f. Prepare for failed intubation.
  2. **Fetal Considerations**
     a. Normal loss of FHR variability and mild bradycardia with general anesthesia.

b. Drugs contraindicated for fetus (e.g., coumadin, verapamil, tetracyclines).
c. In the event of severe maternal trauma or cardiac arrest in which mother's life cannot be saved, an immediate C-section should be performed to save life of fetus who is 24 weeks' gestation or older.
d. Consult high-risk obstetrics service to manage complications best.

Intraoperative Hazards
1. Maternal hypotension with consequent fetal compromise
2. Severe FHR disturbances
3. Precipitation of uterine contractions

Postoperative Problems
1. Postoperative premature contractions
2. Spontaneous abortion
3. Fetal death

SURGICAL PROCEDURE Vaginal Delivery

Objective Termination of pregnancy.

Position
1. Lateral uterine displacement during labor analgesia
2. Lithotomy during actual vaginal delivery

Exposure Perineum.

Incision Episiotomy optional.

Blood Bank Order T&S or none.

Estimated Blood Loss 300 to 500 ml.

Preoperative Studies CBC, platelets, electrolyes, glucose. If patient is preeclamptic, PT, PTT, BUN, creatinine, and fetal scalp blood gas for FHR abnormalities.

Anesthetic Choices Local with IV analgesia; inhalation analgesia; regional technique.
1. IV analgesia; meperidine generally used.
2. Inhalation analgesia requires close monitoring of patient's mental status and ensuring her ability to maintain airway protection.
3. Regional technique, e.g., continuous epidural catheter: caudal or paracervical block for first stage; pudendal block for second stage.

Invasive Monitoring None unless indicated by associated medical conditions. *Preeclampsia management:* Central venous catheter (CVC), Foley, and arterial line are recommended for *severe hypertension.* Pulmonary artery catheter (PAC) is recommended if preeclamptic patient develops *oliguria, congestive heart failure* (CHF), or *complicated hemodynamic abnormality.*

Airway Considerations   See Cesarean Section.

Aspiration Precautions   Always considered full stomach.

Estimated Surgical Time   Average labor time in primipara is 12 hours for first stage and 2 hours for second stage. When fetal head is crowning, it is a matter of minutes to delivery.

Anesthetic Considerations   See Anesthetic Considerations for Cesarean Section. Labor analgesia requires T8 level block (nerves involved in stage 1 are T10–L1, and in stage II are S2–S4). Saddle block needed for vaginal delivery when patient is fully dilated. Equipment for general anesthesia and for neonatal resuscitation should be available. Maintain patient in lateral uterine decubitus position with regional technique if she is hypotensive.

Intraoperative Hazards
1. *Maternal.* Anesthesia-related: e.g., hypotension, local anesthetic toxicity. Non-anesthesia-related: e.g., uterine problems (rupture, inversion); retained placenta; concealed or nonconcealed bleeding; exacerbation of underlying maternal condition, whether gestational or pregestational (e.g., preeclampsia or eclampsia, heart disease decompensation, idiopathic thrombocytopenic purpura). Preeclampsia may not declare itself until labor begins.
2. *Fetal:* Fetal distress; fetal compromise requiring neonatal resuscitation.

Postoperative Problems
1. *Maternal.* uterine atony; bleeding; rupture; retained placenta; perineal tears; CHF in patients with congenital heart disease, as cardiac output and intravascular volume are highest immediately after delivery. Preeclampsia may first be seen or can intensify after delivery.
2. *Neonatal.* Problems may be congenital or acquired.

Postoperative Tests   HCT, Rh blood type of fetus.

SURGICAL PROCEDURE   Vaginal Hysterectomy

Vaginal hysterectomy may have to be abandoned in lieu of an abdominal approach if complications arise.

Objective   Removal of abnormal uterus, rarely with ovaries and tubes. Dilatation and curettage (D&C) precedes hysterectomy.

Position   Lithotomy for D&C; lithotomy with Trendelenburg for hysterectomy.

Exposure   Costal margins to pubis.

Incision   Midline abdominal or transverse suprapubic.

Nerves Involved   Cervical and uterine innervation is from T10–L1 and vaginal innervation is sacral. Therefore level of regional technique must be higher than T10.

Blood Bank Order   T&S.

Estimated Blood Loss   Less than 500 ml.

Preoperative Studies   Routine.

Anesthetic Choices   Spinal, epidural, or general.

Invasive Monitoring   Urinary catheter used to empty bladder at beginning of procedure.

Airway Considerations   Oral endotracheal tube (OETT).

Aspiration Precautions   Not necessary unless an emergency procedure or patient is at risk of gastric reflux.

Estimated Surgical Time   1 to 2 hours.

➤ **Anesthetic Considerations**
1. Positioning injuries
2. Bleeding
3. Patient movement

Intraoperative Hazards
1. Bleeding
2. Injury to bladder, ureter, or rectum
3. Venous air embolism
4. Perioperative thromboembolism

Postoperative Pain Intensity   Mild to moderate.

Postoperative Pain Control   Usually routine parenteral.

REFERENCES
Cesarean Section
Hood DD. Obstetrical Anesthesia Complications and Problems. In Hood DD (ed), Problems in Anesthesia. Philadelphia: J.B. Lippincott, vol. 3, Jan-Mar, 1989.
Ramanathan S. Obstetric Anesthesia. Philadelphia: Lea & Febiger, 1988.
Shnider SM, Levinson G. Anesthesia for Cesarean Section. In Shnider S, Levinson G (eds), Anesthesia for Obstetrics. Baltimore: Williams & Wilkins, 1993.

Dilatation and Curettage

White PF. Outpatient Anesthesia. In Miller RD (ed), Anesthesia. New York: Churchill Livingstone, 1990.

Laparoscopic Surgery

Peterson HB, Hulka JF, Spielman FJ, Lee S, Murchbanks PA. Local Versus General Anesthesia for Laparoscopic Sterilization: A Randomized Study. Obstet Gynecol 70:903, 1987.

Spielman F. Laparoscopic Surgery. In Hood DD (ed), Problems in Anesthesia. Philadelphia: J.B. Lippincott, vol 3, Jan-Mar 1989.

Nonobstetric Anesthesia for Pregnant Patient

Levinson G, Shnider S. Anesthesia for Surgery during Pregnancy. In Shnider S, Levinson G (eds), Anesthesia for Obstetrics. Baltimore: Williams & Wilkins, 1993.

Ramanathan S. Anesthesia in Non-Obstetric Situations. In Obstetric Anesthesia. Philadelphia: Lea & Febiger, 1988.

Vaginal Delivery

Cohen S. Inhalational Analgesia and Anesthesia for Vaginal Delivery. In Shnider S, Levinson G (eds), Anesthesia for Obstetrics. Baltimore: Williams & Wilkins, 1993.

CHAPTER 8

ORAL AND MAXILLOFACIAL SURGERY

SURGICAL PROCEDURE Dental Surgery

Includes removal of nonrestorable, infected, or impacted teeth, trimming of alveolar bone, and enucleation of odontogenic cysts and tumors. Performed by oral or maxillofacial surgeons.

Objective Incision and drainage for odontogenic infection.

Position Supine.

Exposure Intraoral or extraoral approach.

Incision
1. Transmucosal for intraoral approach and dentoalveolar surgery
2. Extraoral through skin over fluctuant area

Preoperative Studies Routine plus coagulation profile.

Blood Bank Order None.

Estimated Blood Loss Usually minimal.

Anesthetic Choices Local, nerve block, or general. IV sedation or N_2O or both often used at dental offices for minor surgical procedures.

Invasive Monitoring None.

Airway Considerations
1. Airway compromise due to diffuse swelling or infection (e.g., Ludwig's angina from odontogenic infection).
2. Laryngoscopy may rupture abscess or damage tooth with associated poor dentition. Oral intubation is preferable in patients with coagulopathy and cardiac valve disease (bacterial seeding). Otherwise, nasal intubation preferable (blind or under direct visualization; apneic or spontaneously breathing).

Aspiration Precautions   Full stomach if nonelective surgery; emergence should be considered full stomach because of blood's pooling in stomach.

Queries for Surgeon
1. Nasal or oral intubation?
2. Side of oral ETT taping?
3. Extent of surgery planned?

Estimated Surgical Time   Usually less than 1 hour.

➤ Anesthetic Considerations
1. Short procedure.
2. With general anesthetic, consider nasal versus oral endotracheal intubation.
3. Pharyngeal pack use.
4. Use of local anesthetic and epinephrine.
5. Inaccessibility of head and long extension tubing set-up on ventilator circuit.
6. Head-up position to decrease blood loss.

Conventional anesthetic is suited for outpatient procedure. Goal is rapid recovery with patient readiness for postoperative home discharge, i.e., control of pain, nausea, and vomiting and relatively alert mental status. Routine antinausea measures (e.g., pharyngeal pack, suctioning stomach, pharmacotherapy) are useful. Ensure pharyngeal pack removal by surgeon at end of the procedure.

Intraoperative Hazards
1. Endotracheal tube (ETT) displacement during general anesthesia
2. Aspiration of blood or purulent material

Postoperative Problems
1. Hematoma formation
2. Bacteremia
3. Bleeding
4. Aspiration
5. Foreign body causing obstruction
6. Laryngospasm
7. Endocarditis from bacterial seeding from nasal intubation or dental procedure

Postoperative Pain Intensity   Moderate.

Postoperative Pain Control   Oral acetaminophen and codeine or other nonsteroidal antiinflammatory drug such as ketorolac tromethamine (Toradol).

SURGICAL PROCEDURE Mandibular Surgery

Includes sagittal split osteotomy, mandibular osteotomy, repair of mandibular fractures, mandibular resection and reconstruction, orthognathic surgery, temporomandibular joint (TMJ) reconstruction, and vestibuloplasty. Intermaxillary fixation (IMF)—the fastening of upper teeth to lower teeth with elastic bands or wires—is common to most of these procedures.

Position Supine.

Blood Bank Order T&C 2 units PRBCs.

Estimated Blood Loss Variable. Osteotomies may incur 500–1000 ml blood loss.

Preoperative Studies Routine and coagulation profile.

Anesthetic Choice General.

Invasive Monitoring None.

Airway Considerations
1. Nasal endotracheal tube (ETT), e.g., nasal RAE tube, for IMF.
2. If mouth opening is limited only because of trismus, e.g., mandibular fracture, may use paralysis for endotracheal intubation (ETI). However, if mouth opening is limited for anatomic reasons, TMJ fracture or TMJ disease, maintain spontaneous respiration for ETI because of potential for difficult airway.
3. Nasal ETI can be performed with spontaneous ventilation, with paralysis, blind, or with laryngoscopy. Topical anesthesia with vasoconstrictor (Neosynephrine) and lidocaine or just cocaine recommended prior to nasal ETI.
4. Ketamine (plus an antisialagogue, e.g., glycopyrrolate 0.2 mg IV) useful for spontaneously breathing, sedated intubation.

Aspiration Precautions Not necessary unless an emergency procedure or patient is at risk of gastric reflux.

Estimated Surgical Time 2 to 3 hours.

➤ **Anesthetic Considerations**
1. **Preoperative Considerations**
   Most important is airway.
2. **Anesthetic Considerations**
   a. Airway considerations mentioned above.
   b. No access to head and neck.
   c. Pharyngeal pack sometimes used.
   d. Nerve stimulation by surgeon sometimes required; therefore degree of paralysis should be >1 to 2 twitches on train-of-four (TOF).
   e. Close, continuous monitoring of ventilation (e.g., precordial stethoscope) for ETT displacement or kinking.
   f. Mandibular reconstruction may require bone or nerve grafts.

3. Anesthetic Technique
a. Ensure secure tube attachment and eye protection.
b. Place extensions on breathing circuit and on IV tubing. Surgeons are working in the same space.
c. Antinausea measures recommended.
d. Ensure pharyngeal pack removal by surgeon at end of procedure before IMF.
e. Extubation generally performed in postanesthesia recovery room to ensure alert, responsive patient with adequate neuromuscular function, gas exchange, and control of nausea and vomiting.

Intraoperative Hazards
1. ETT displacement
2. Bleeding
3. Risk of nasal trauma or bleeding with ETT
4. Pneumothorax from rib graft for TMJ reconstruction

Postoperative Management   PACU with intubation.

Postoperative Problems
1. Airway compromise due to laryngospasm
2. Airway obstruction
3. Vomiting or respiratory depression
   Comments: Wire cutter should be available at bedside at all times, since postextubation laryngospasm or vomiting with IMF is problematic and may require immediate release of IMF.

Postoperative Pain Intensity   Moderate.

Postoperative Pain Control   PCA, routine parenteral narcotics.

SURGICAL PROCEDURE   Maxillary Surgery

Includes maxillary fractures, major resections or reconstructions, Le Fort I osteotomy, zygomatic fractures. Maxillary fractures are classified as Le Fort I, II, or III, with Le Fort III involving complete craniofacial dissociation.

Preoperative Studies   HCT; depend on suspected underlying conditions or injuries; may also include toxicology screen.

Blood Bank Order   T&C 2 units PRBCs.

Estimated Blood Loss   Large: high vascularity of facial area.

Anesthetic Choices   General anesthesia. Le Fort III fractures are a contraindication to nasal intubation since they are often associated with basal skull fractures and nasal intubation could result in intracranial intubation. Skull CT or MRI would be required to rule out basal skull fracture.

Airway Considerations
1. Difficult airway.
2. Procedures involving intermaxillary fixation (IMF) require nasal endotracheal intubation (ETI).
3. Stabilize trauma patient's neck before manipulation if neck fracture has not been ruled out.
4. Airway may be difficult to intubate or may be compromised by traumatic anatomic distortion, edema, or bleeding.
5. Patient requiring reconstruction for congenital facial deformity may have associated congenital heart disease, e.g., Down syndrome.
6. Facial fractures may compromise airway and require emergency intervention. Worst case scenario, i.e., oral and nasal trauma, may require emergency cricothyroidotomy.

Aspiration Precautions None unless an emergency procedure or patient is at risk of gastric reflux.

Queries for Surgeon
1. Use of IMF?
2. Projected blood loss?
3. Nerve stimulation?
4. Tracheostomy?

Estimated Surgical Time Variable.

➤ Anesthetic Considerations
1. **Preoperative Considerations**
   a. Associated injuries, especially neck and intracranial injuries.
   b. Underlying medical condition that caused the accident, e.g., Stokes-Adams attack, transient ischemic attack (TIA), or drug intoxication resulting in motor vehicle crash.
2. **Anesthetic Problems**
   a. Airway may be difficult.
   b. Endotracheal tube (ETT) type: RAE (preformed) tube, armored tube, or nasal tube often used. Tracheostomy may be required in major procedures. Maxillary reconstructions and fracture repair and nonzygomatic fracture require IMF and therefore nasal intubations.
   c. Use of pharyngeal packs.
   d. Surgical procedure may involve bone (e.g., rib or iliac crest) or nerve graft (e.g., dural nerve) harvest.
   e. Surgical infiltration of epinephrine should be limited to <5 µg/kg in children undergoing halothane anesthesia (i.e., 1 ml/kg 1:200,000 solution).
   f. Inaccessibility of head.

Intraoperative Hazards
1. Complication of nasal tubes: ETT or nasogastric tube into cranium or inadvertent ETT displacement (extubation or endobronchial)
2. Major blood loss
3. Pneumothorax with rib graft
4. Arrhythmias with epinephrine and halothane

Postoperative Problems
1. Airway
2. Bleeding
3. CSF leak
4. Nausea and vomiting in patient with IMF
5. Timing of extubation

Postoperative Pain Intensity   Moderate.

Postoperative Pain Control   Parenteral narcotics.

SURGICAL PROCEDURE   Salivary Gland Surgery

Includes parotidectomy and excision of sublingual gland and submandibular gland.

Objective   Removal of salivary glands is indicated for tumors, cysts, chronic infection, chronic obstruction, or some inflammatory processes.

Position   Supine with or without thyroid bag for neck extension.

Incision   Similar to that for face lift: mostly hidden in creases.

Preoperative Studies   Routine; HCT and coagulation profile.

Estimated Blood Loss   Little. Major loss rare.

Anesthetic Choice   General anesthesia. Nasotracheal intubation preferred.

Invasive Monitoring   None.

Airway Considerations   Difficult airway may be expected in cases of airway distortion from tumors or cysts. Postoperative edema or hematoma formation may compromise airway.

Aspiration Precautions   None unless urgent surgery for infection or patient is at risk of gastric reflux.

Queries for Surgeon
1. Side of endotracheal tube (ETT) taping?
2. Preference for type of ETT (e.g., RAE tube)?
3. Major blood loss expected?

Estimated Surgical Time   1 to 2 hours.

➤ **Anesthetic Considerations**
1. Don't paralyze without consulting the surgeon because of potential for 7th nerve injury and occasional need for 7th nerve stimulation.
2. No head and neck access intraoperatively.
3. Type of ETT, e.g., nasal RAE tube or reinforced tube.

4. Use of pharyngeal packs in sublingual gland removal.
5. Emesis due to blood collected in stomach requires full stomach considerations on emergence.

Intraoperative Hazards
1. ETT displacement or kinking
2. Bleeding

Postoperative Problem   Airway compromise due to bleeding, hematoma, or edema.

Postoperative Pain Intensity   Moderate.

Postoperative Pain Control   Oral or parenteral narcotics.

Postoperative Tests   Coagulation profile; HCT optional.

SUGGESTED READING
Dental Surgery
Orkin FK, Gold B. Selection. In Wetchler B (ed), Anesthesia for Ambulatory Surgery. Philadelphia: J.B. Lippincott, 1991.
White PF. Outpatient Anesthesia. In Miller RD (ed), Anesthesia. New York: Churchill Livingstone, 1990.

Mandibular Surgery
Davies RM, Scott JG. Anesthesia for Major Oral and Maxillofacial Surgery. Br J Anaesth 40:202, 1968.
Gotta A, Sullivan CA. Anesthetic Management of Maxillofacial Trauma. In McGoldrich KM (ed), Anesthesia for Ophthalmic and Otolaryngologic Surgery. Philadelphia: W.B. Saunders, 1992.

CHAPTER 9

ORTHOPEDIC PROCEDURES

SURGICAL PROCEDURE Hemipelvectomy (Internal or Complete)

Objective To reduce morbidity and mortality from a severely damaged, diseased, or tumor-ridden pelvic or proximal femoral segment. For internal hemipelvectomy, bony parts and some musculature are removed. As long as the sciatic nerve and femoral artery vein and nerve are retained, limb can be useful. In complete hemipelvectomy, entire lower extremity is removed along with the hemipelvis.

Position Lateral decubitus position (Fig. 2). Occasionally with patient supine but tilted at 45-degree angle with head up.

Exposure Below knee to the lower ribs and across the midline both anteriorly and posteriorly. The exposed region, draped free, usually includes upper thigh, both midlines, and lower ribs.

Incision Along iliac crest and around the thigh.

Blood Bank Order T&C 8 units PRBCs. Autologous techniques (i.e., cell saver, predonation, hemodilution) useful; controlled hypotensive technique optional.

Estimated Blood Loss Can be massive. Complete hemipelvectomy entails less blood loss than internal hemipelvectomy does, since the common iliac artery can be ligated early.

Preoperative Studies CBC, coagulation profile, electrolytes, BUN, creatinine, glucose; others as indicated.

Anesthetic Choices General anesthesia alone or with regional technique (optional).

Invasive Monitoring Arterial lines, Foley catheter; CVP monitoring is important because of massive fluid requirements and ureteral disruption.

Airway Considerations Routine.

Aspiration Precautions   Not necessary unless an emergency procedure or patient is at risk of gastric reflux.

Estimated Surgical Time   Prolonged; 8 to 12 hours.

➤ **Anesthetic Considerations**
1. **Preoperative Evaluation**
   Complicated by an oncology patient population or platelet dysfunction due to use of anti-inflammatory agents. Since loss of limb may be emotionally taxing, preoperative visit and sedation are mandatory.
2. **Anesthetic Problems**
   a. Lengthy procedure.
   b. Major blood loss. Requires two large-bore IV accesses, invasive monitoring, hypothermia-prevention measures, and availability of sufficient blood. Major site of bleeding is internal iliac artery.
   c. Inability to assess urinary output because of ureteral disruption.
   d. Maintenance of patient in one position for a prolonged period.
   e. Postoperative and phantom-limb pain.

Postoperative Management   ICU if massive transfusions required.

Postoperative Pain Intensity   Severe.

Postoperative Pain Control   Parenteral narcotics, PCA, regional.

SURGICAL PROCEDURE   Hip Surgery

Includes (1) total hip replacement, (2) internal fixation of hip for fracture, and (3) hip arthrodesis.

Objectives
1. Total hip replacement: To relieve pain and improve function in an arthritic hip or a hip badly damaged by osteonecrosis or tumor.
2. Internal fixation of hip for fracture: To stabilize the fracture of the neck of the femur or intertrochanteric region.
3. Hip arthrodesis: To relieve pain, diminish disability, correct alignment, and improve gait.

Positions
1. Total hip replacement: Usually lateral decubitus position (Fig. 2). Some surgeons prefer an anterior approach with patient supine.
2. Internal fixation of hip for fracture: Patient supine on fracture table (Fig. 1).
3. Hip arthrodesis: Supine, with a pad beneath the buttock of the affected side.

Exposure   From lower ribcage to midthigh.

Incisions
1. Total hip replacement: Long incision paralleling the femoral shaft.
2. Internal fixation of hip fracture: 5 cm incision over lateral side of the proximal thigh in the region of trochanter.
3. Hip arthrodesis: Along the lateral aspect of the hip region and the trochanter and down the shaft.

Blood Bank Order T&C 2 units PRBCs. Controlled hypotensive technique; autotransfusion techniques optional.

Estimated Blood Loss 500 to 1000 ml during the procedure. Hip fractures sometimes associated with loss of over 1000 ml of blood before patient arrives in OR. Intraoperatively, blood loss may exceed 1000 ml, especially with redo or complicated procedures. Postoperatively, hematocrit may fall because of concealed bleeding within tissues.

Preoperative Studies CBC, coagulation profile, electrolytes, glucose, creatinine, ECG. For trauma or elderly patients, further preoperative workup may be necessary.

Anesthetic Choices General anesthesia with endotracheal intubation, epidural, continuous spinal or single-shot spinal.

Nerves Involved L1–S2 nerve roots or femoral nerve, lateral femoral cutaneous, sciatic nerve, and obturator nerve.

Invasive Monitoring Arterial line optional; CVP helpful but optional.

Airway Considerations Routine.

Aspiration Precautions Trauma or emergency patients, as well as patients at risk of gastric reflux, need to be assessed as if the stomach were full.

Estimated Surgical Time 2 to 4 hours.

➤ **Anesthetic Considerations**
1. **Preoperative Evaluation**
   Complicated: often elderly, arthritic, patients taking steroids or NSAIDs; trauma patients. Preoperative evaluation and optimization should take into account that dislocated hips are an emergency procedure and that patients with hip fractures are at increasing risk of thromboembolic disease with delays in surgery. Selection of anesthetic technique depends on patient preference and on the patient's ability to cooperate and to tolerate being maintained in one position for the time required for major orthopedic surgery.
2. **Anesthetic Problems**
   a. Position: Conscious patients become uncomfortable and agitated in lateral decubitus position on a fracture table.
   b. Pain during positioning for placement of regional anesthesia can be eased with narcotics or ketamine or both.
   c. Causes for induction of general anesthesia during regional anesthesia include wearing off of regional, an inadequate regional, an uncooperative patient, or cardiorespiratory decompensation. Intubation of pa-

tient in lateral position is easier if he is in left lateral decubitus; however, with assistance, induction and intubation may be easily achieved even when the patient is in the right lateral decubitus position.
   d. Methylmethacrylate, which is used to stabilize the hip prosthesis, produces a transient drop in blood pressure and hypoxemia that is accentuated in hypovolemia. This can be counteracted with adequate replenishment of circulating blood volume.
   e. Advantages of regional anesthesia over general anesthesia: Decreased stress response, respiratory benefits such as less $\dot{V}/\dot{Q}$ mismatch, reduced incidence of venous thromboembolism, and postoperative analgesia.
   f. Blood loss and hypothermia.
3. **Anesthetic Technique**
   a. Routine monitoring.
   b. Large-bore IV access.
   c. Conventional general anesthetic or regional.
   d. Controlled hypotension can be used to decrease blood loss; arterial line is required for controlled hypotension.
   e. Prevention of hypothermia.
   f. Perioperative antibiotics.
   g. Relaxation with muscle paralysis helps surgeon.

Postoperative Pain Intensity   Moderate.

Postoperative Pain Control   Regional, PCA, parenteral narcotics.

SURGICAL PROCEDURE   Lower Extremity

Includes tibial, fibular, knee, ankle, and foot procedures.

Objectives
1. Open reductions and internal fixation
2. Tumor resection
3. Relief of compartment syndromes
4. Diagnostic and therapeutic arthroscopic surgery of the knee
5. Lower extremity amputation
6. Achilles tendon repair

Position   Most often supine (Fig. 1).

Exposure   Extremity draped free. Prepped toes to groin or lower.

Blood Bank Order   Most often T&C 2 units PRBCs. None for minor surgery such as arthroscopy and foot procedures.

Estimated Blood Loss   Limited by tourniquet use. May be extensive in tumor resections.

Preoperative Studies   Routine, plus as indicated.

Anesthetic Choices   General or regional.
1. General anesthesia with mask, laryngeal mask, or endotracheal intubation.
2. Regional may involve spinal, epidural, or "3 in 1" block: sciatic-femoral block, lumbar plexus block, popliteal block, ankle block, digital block, or IV Bier block.
3. Features of various blocks:
    a. Spinal: Dense, rapid block but hemodynamic changes are a possibility; contraindicated in patient with significant coagulopathy. Risk of postdural puncture headache.
    b. Epidural: More gentle onset of block; continuous catheter technique is advantageous because level and duration of anesthesia are easy to control. Disadvantages are slower onset, sympathectomy, contraindication in coagulopathy, and risk of postdural puncture headache.
    c. Major nerve blocks. Major benefit is lack of significant hemodynamic changes. Disadvantages: It is less reliable and is a complete block.
    d. IV regional or Bier block, e.g., for foot or ankle procedures. Advantages are that there is no sympathectomy and no postdural puncture headaches.

Invasive Monitoring   Generally none. May be indicated in trauma patients, critically ill patients, or patients in whom major fluid shifts are expected (e.g., some tumor resections).

Airway Considerations   Assess airway carefully in arthritic patient (cervical spine arthritis involvement).

Aspiration Precautions   Use aspiration precautions with trauma patients.

➤ **Anesthetic Considerations**
1. **Preoperative Evaluation**
    Routine evaluation but pay special attention to trauma patients for associated injuries, hemodynamic status, and intoxication status; oncology-associated medical problems; hematologic status (namely coagulation profile); IV access; arthritic patients' airways.
2. **Anesthetic Goals**
    Goals include providing patient comfort and safe positioning; monitoring for blood loss; and monitoring and informing surgeon of tourniquet time.
3. **Anesthetic Problems**
    a. Use of C-arm fluoroscopy and exposure to radiation. Wear lead shielding.
    b. Tourniquet pain.
    c. Inadequate blocks requiring additional block, IV sedation, N_2O or general anesthesia.
    d. Complications of procedure such as fat emboli and neurovascular injury.

Postoperative Pain Intensity   Moderate to severe.

Postoperative Pain Control   Regional local anesthetic, spinal opioids, PCA, IV narcotics, routine.

SURGICAL PROCEDURE Lumbar Laminectomy (with or without Arthrodesis)

Performed mostly for removal of herniated disk or to relieve vertebral stenosis.

Objective Laminectomy may involve simple resection of lamina of single vertebral segment all the way to almost complete resection of posterior elements of two or more segments. An extensive arthrodesis requires use of local bone (iliac crest).

Position Prone (Fig. 4). Occasionally lateral decubitus is used (Fig. 2). Various frames are used for prone position. Goals are to allow free abdominal excursion, to decrease venous engorgement in lower body, and to diminish lumbar lordosis.

Exposure Vertebral and paravertebral regions; posterior aspect of iliac crest is optional.

Incision Midline back; 5 to 15 cm incision is made, depending on the number of levels to be explored. Degree of bony lamina, joint, and pedicle removal depends on the extent of the process. For *simple discectomy* a hemilaminectomy is carried out. Microscope may be used. For *spinal stenosis* a two-level or more laminectomy involving removal of the lateral joints and facets as well may be necessary. *Laminectomy for tumors* extends above and below the level of the tumor. Exact site of operation may require intraoperative roentgenologic verification.

Blood Bank Order T&C 2 units PRBCs.

Estimated Blood Loss 400 ml.

Preoperative Studies HCT and coagulation profile, plus any others indicated by patient's medical history.

Anesthetic Choices General anesthetic most commonly used; regional (spinal) rarely used. Postoperative analgesia can be offered by a spinal narcotic (e.g., morphine sulfate 0.3–0.5 mg) administered intraoperatively by the surgeon while there is direct dural exposure and patient is under general anesthesia.

Invasive Monitoring Routine. Foley is mandatory for lengthy procedures.

Airway Considerations None.

Aspiration Precautions None.

Estimated Surgical Time 2 to 3 hours.

➤ **Anesthetic Considerations**
  1. **Preoperative Evaluation**
     Pay special attention to associated medical problems and neurologic deficits.
  2. **Anesthetic Problems**
     a. Positioning. Prone position is associated with respiratory compromise and decreased venous return, especially when abdominal excursions are hindered. Postinduction hemodynamic sag is common after patient is turned. Positioning-related injuries are possible. Pay special attention to eyes, ears, breasts, genitalia, and brachial plexus. Straighten arms by patient's side when turning him. (See Prone position, Fig. 4.)
     b. Blood loss usually is not extensive with laminectomy. Depends on extent of procedure, surgeon's skill, and anesthetic technique with respect to use of controlled hypotension and proper positioning. Increased abdominal pressure increases vertebral venous blood loss.
     c. Other hazards. Accidental extubation or cardiac arrest in prone position requires immediate turning of patient back to supine position. Venous air embolism is rare.
  3. **Anesthetic Technique**
     a. General anesthetic.
     b. Intubate patient on stretcher before transfer to OR table.
     c. Intubation could be performed in awake patient by neuroleptanalgesia technique to facilitate positioning.
     d. *Maintenance.* Assure immobility, especially during surgical dissection around nerve roots.
     e. *Emergence.* Patient is generally extubated after being turned supine onto stretcher. Extubation in prone patient possible if he is awake, responsive, fully reversed, and breathing spontaneously and did not have a difficult airway.

Intraoperative Hazards
  1. Fat embolism.
  2. Movement because of inadequate depth of anesthesia or inadequate paralysis.
  3. Compression injuries: pressure sores, supraorbital nerve palsies, and blindness.
  4. Endotracheal tube and IV line displacement during turning.
  5. Accidental extubation of patient in prone position would require reintubation with patient supine.
  6. Shoulder dislocation is possible if patient is paralyzed when being turned.

Postoperative Problems Patients are required to remain supine or with head up at a 30-degree angle, thus promoting atelectasis and desaturation after extubation. Check neurologic integrity especially of lower extremities immediately after surgery.

Postoperative Pain Intensity Moderate to severe.

Postoperative Pain Control Routine, PCA, spinal opioids.

SURGICAL PROCEDURE Scoliosis

Scoliosis is a lateral curvature of the spine associated with deformity of the vertebrae and rib cage. The thoracic and lumbar spines are involved most frequently. Severity is related to the angle of scoliosis or Cobb's angle. Posterior spinal fusion using Harrington rods is the corrective procedure most often performed. Correction is indicated when Cobb's angle is >50 degrees. Cause of 75% of cases is unknown. Cases of unknown cause occur predominantly in teenage girls. Known causes include neuromuscular and myopathic disease and trauma.

Objective Correct lateral curvature of rib cage to halt decline in respiratory function.

Position Prone (Fig. 4).

Exposure Back.

Incision Midline back.

Blood Bank Order T&C 4 units PRBCs; autologous predonation or autotransfusion or both are recommended.

Estimated Blood Loss Can be >10 units.

Preoperative Studies HCT, ABGs, CXR, PFTs.

Anesthetic Choices General; hypotensive techniques optional. Use of regional technique possible. With controlled hypotension the risk of spinal cord ischemia increases.

Invasive Monitoring Foley catheter, arterial line; central venous catheter and somatosensory-evoked potential (SSEPs) are optional.

Airway Considerations Airway can be difficult and require fiberoptic intubation, especially in severe kyphoscoliosis.

Aspiration Precautions Standard considerations.

Queries for Surgeon Intraoperative wake-up test?

Estimated Surgical Time 4 to 6 hours.

➤ **Anesthetic Considerations**
 1. **Preoperative Evaluation or Optimization**
    Routine history, physical examination, and laboratory studies. Pay special attention to:
    a. Pediatric age group.
    b. Underlying cause, such as neuromuscular disease with associated respiratory muscle weakness.
    c. Associated medical problems. Respiratory disease (chronic hypoxia, restrictive pulmonary disease), secondary pulmonary hypertension, or

cor pulmonale and right-sided heart failure. Check PFTs, CXR, and ABGs as minimum baseline investigations. Patient may require pre-operative pulmonary and cardiovascular optimization.

    d. Informed consent includes:

       (1) Procedure

       (2) Anesthetic technique

       (3) Anesthetic risks

       (4) Invasive monitoring

       (5) Wake-up test and risk of recall

       (6) Possible postoperative ventilation and ICU admission

       (7) Potential for homologous blood transfusion

2. Anesthetic Problems

    a. Pediatric anesthetic considerations.

    b. Prone position with consequent respiratory compromise, cardiovascular compromise, compression injuries to eyes, face, breasts, genitals, groins; risks during turning of patient. Anesthesia induced with patient on stretcher. Patient turns and positions on his own from stretcher to OR table (after neuroleptic-type intubation) or with assistance.

    c. Blood loss can be extensive.

    d. Temperature is unstable during prolonged procedure.

    e. Spinal cord function testing:

       (1) **Wake-up test:** Patient is awakened during procedure, regardless of the anesthetic technique used and is asked to move his lower extremities. Patient is then put back to sleep. Problems can require reversal of relaxant and narcotics, leading to intraoperative recall and agitation and sudden movement.

       (2) SSEPs monitor integrity of dorsal columns. Problems with SSEPs are such that a constant level of anesthesia is required and the anterior cord (motor function) cannot be monitored. In the event of loss of SSEP, optimize BP, lighten inhalation anesthesia, loosen distraction on rods, and perform wake-up test if integrity of cord is still a concern.

    f. Other intraoperative problems include risk of pneumothorax with thoracic scoliosis procedures; risk of venous air embolism due to large venous sinuses within paraspinal region; and associated neuromuscular diseases, scoliosis, and malignant hyperthermia.

Postoperative Management   PACU; possibly ICU.

Postoperative Problems   Mostly pulmonary related. Neurologic spinal cord deficit occurs in 1% of cases.

Postoperative Pain Intensity   Moderate to severe.

Postoperative Pain Control   Parenteral narcotics, PCA.

Postoperative Tests   HCT, ABGs, CXR, neurologic testing of lower extremities immediately after wake-up.

SURGICAL PROCEDURE Upper Extremity

Includes upper extremity amputations, operations on the shoulder, elbow, forearm, hands, and wrist.

Position Most often supine (Fig. 1).

Exposure Upper extremity.

Blood Bank Order Orders for shoulder and arm procedures and those for trauma patients generally are to T&C 2 units PRBCs. With more distal procedures, no order necessary.

Estimated Blood Loss Greatest with shoulder procedure (e.g., shoulder arthrodesis, upper extremity amputations); least with elective distal procedures.

Preoperative Studies Routine plus as indicated.

Anesthetic Choices General, regional, or local. General with mask, laryngeal mask, or endotracheal tube. Several options exist for regional technique. Brachial plexus block can be used for any of the surgical procedures of the upper extremity including shoulder procedures (shoulder procedures may require supraspinatus nerve block as well). Brachial plexus block involves large volume of anesthetic (30–40 ml). There are three brachial plexus blocks: (1) interscalene, (2) supraclavicular or perivascular, and (3) axillary. *Disadvantages* of brachial plexus block:
1. Interscalene often provides inadequate ulnar block.
2. Supraclavicular or perivascular provides the most complete block of the brachial plexus but carries greatest risk of pneumothorax.
3. Axillary inadequately blocks musculocutaneous nerve (which provides sensory innervation to lateral forearm and motor innervation to biceps) and intercostal brachial nerve (medial arm) and sometimes allows only poor control of tourniquet pain.

Wrist blocks, digital blocks, and IV regional are useful for more distal procedures.

Invasive Monitoring None.

Airway Considerations Routine.

Aspiration Precautions Present in trauma procedures or if patient is at risk of gastric reflux.

Queries for Surgeon Estimated duration of procedure?

➤ **Anesthetic Considerations**
  1. **Preoperative Evaluation**
     Routine evaluation plus special attention to associated conditions in acute trauma patients (intoxication, hypovolemia, cervical spine associated injuries).

2. **Anesthetic Problems**
   a. Selection of patient for regional.
   b. Microvascular and reimplantation procedures could take >12 hours. Regional requires continuous catheter technique. Other issues are positioning, patient's discomfort, temperature monitoring, humidified gases, and avoiding N_2O for procedures that take longer than 12 hours. Prolonged N_2O may suppress bone marrow function.
   c. Tourniquet pain is common even with general anesthesia. BP will begin to progressively rise 30 minutes after the procedure has begun.

Intraoperative Hazards
1. Local anesthetic toxicity.
2. Neurovascular injury related to block.
3. Inadequate regional. May require salvaging technique ("rescue block" at level of elbow, wrist, or fingers), additional local, IV sedation, or general anesthesia.
4. Tourniquet pain.
5. Patient movement during microvascular procedure.

Postoperative Pain Control Regional block, PCA, IV narcotics, routine.

SUGGESTED READINGS
Bernstein RZ, Rosenberg AD. Anesthesia for Orthopedic Surgery. Semin Anesth 4:36-43, 1987.
Smith T. Anesthesia and Orthopedic Surgery. In Barash P (ed), Clinical Anesthesiology. London: J.B. Lippincott, 1992.

CHAPTER 10

PEDIATRIC AND NEONATAL PROCEDURES

SURGICAL PROCEDURE General Pediatric Considerations

Airway Considerations The child's airway is different from that of the adult because of large head, large tongue, long and stiff epiglottis, cephalad larynx, and narrow and short trachea. The cricoid is the narrowest point. Children <3 months old are obligate nasal breathers. Use uncuffed endotracheal tube (ETT) in children <8 years old to decrease resistance and prevent postoperative stridor.

Respiratory System Children desaturate quickly, and anesthesia is rapidly induced by inhalation technique because of increased minute ventilation and decreased functional residual capacity (FRC). Infants and young children require controlled ventilation (as opposed to spontaneous ventilation) because they have compliant chest wall, proportionately fewer fatigue-resistant respiratory muscle fibers, greater sensitivity to anesthetic agents, and increased oxygen consumption. In children <10 kg nonrebreathing circuit (Mapleson D or Bain) often used. Advantages of the nonrebreathing circuit are low resistance (no valves), decreased dead space, light weight, and easy to feel changes in respiratory system compliance.

Cardiovascular System Cardiac output is dependent on heart rate because of stiffness of left ventricle and fixed stroke volume. Hypovolemia decreases BP much sooner than it does in an adult.

Fluids Ringer's lactate is recommended for maintenance in the older child and for replacement of third space losses in all children. Younger children and infants have little ability to handle fluid or electrolyte abnormalities: they are unable to handle too much or too little Na, K^+, or free water. They require administration and monitoring of glucose because of their high metabolic rate and low glycogen stores. Therefore, $D_{2.5}$ to D_5 in 0.2 to 0.5 NS with 20 mEq/L of KCl is recommended as maintenance for infants.

Idiosyncratic Reactions to Anesthetics
1. Halothane hepatitis virtually unheard of in pediatrics.
2. Incidence of malignant hyperthermia higher in pediatrics. Dantrolene needs to be readily available.

Temperature Instability Infants are more prone to hypothermia because of their large body-surface-area-to-weight ratio, lack of shivering thermogenesis, lack of subcutaneous fat, and immature thermoregulatory CNS center.

Psychiatric Considerations
1. Infants 0 to 6 months old are unaffected by short separation from parents and thus do not require preoperative sedation.
2. Children 6 months to 4 years old have maximum psychological disturbance and varying degrees of suspicion of strangers, especially in 2 year olds ("terrible twos").
3. Children 4 to 12 years old have fear of bodily harm and are more logical. Young adolescents may exhibit some emotional lability and fear loss of control. Older teens are more concerned about bodily mutilation.

Fasting Guidelines Conventionally NPO for milk and solids 4 to 6 hours before surgery.
1. Infants 0 to 6 months old: clear fluids offered 2 hours before surgery or have IV started for maintenance fluid administration preoperatively.
2. Infants >6 months old: clear fluids 3 hours before surgery.

Monitoring Routine monitoring in order of importance:
1. Anesthesia personnel at all times are most important monitor.
2. SaO_2, precordial or esophageal stethoscope, ECG leads, BP cuff, temperature monitor.
3. $ETCO_2$, although less accurate and more cumbersome in infants.
4. Transcutaneous PO_2 generally not used in OR.
5. Arterial line, central venous catheter, and Foley if necessary.
6. Pulmonary artery catheter rarely used in children.

Equipment Pediatric size endotracheal tube (ETT), laryngoscope, mask and oral airway, breathing circuit, ventilator, breathing bag, BP cuff, fluid bags, IV lines, Foley catheter, esophageal or precordial stethoscope, ECG pads, SaO_2 probe.

Miscellaneous Guidelines
1. ETT size (ID) for child >2 years old: (Age in years/4) + 4.
2. ETT length (cm) for child >2 years old = 11 + (Age/2)
3. Maximum allowable blood loss = Blood volume × [HCT (measured) − HCT (desired)]/HCT measured.
4. Maintenance fluid requirements:
   0-10 kg: 100 ml/kg/d or 4 ml/kg/h
   10-20 kg: 50 ml/kg/d or 2 ml/kg/h
   >20 kg: 20 ml/kg/d or 1 ml/kg/h
   (e.g., 40 kg:1000 + 500 + 400 = 1900 ml/d; or 40 kg: 40 + 20 + 20 = 80 ml/h)
5. Fresh gas flows needed to maintain eucapnia on nonrebreathing circuit such as a Mapleson D are 2 to 3 times minute ventilation on spontaneous breathing and on controlled ventilation. Nonrebreathing circuits are rec-

ommended only for children <10 kg because of their lower resistance and dead space, although circle system can also be used in controlled ventilation. Heated humidification is recommended in either system.

6. Fresh gas flows need not be increased on circle system because of CO_2 absorber.

7. Respiratory parameters: tidal volumes are approximately 8 to 10 ml/kg, although can be adjusted based on visual inspection of child's chest. Rate is approximately 40/min for neonates, 20 to 30/min for 1 year old, and 20/min for 4 year old.

8. N.B: Acceptable systolic BP is 60 mm Hg for neonate and >70 mm Hg for 1 year old.

➤ **Anesthetic Considerations**
Pediatric
1. **Preoperative Evaluation Goals**
   a. Evaluate medical status of patient.
   b. Allay patient's and parents' anxieties.
   c. Order premedication if necessary. (IM atropine no longer administered routinely before surgery.)

2. **Induction**
   Intubation performed with child either awake (sick neonate or child with difficult airway) or asleep with or without muscle relaxant.
   a. Hypnosis
      (1) PO (e.g., triclofos 75 mg/kg 1½ to 2 hours before surgery or midazolam 0.5 to 1.0 mg/kg dissolved in sweet syrup).
      (2) IM (e.g., pentobarbital or secobarbital 4 mg/kg 1½ to 2 hours before surgery or ketamine 4 to 10 mg, which takes effect in 3 to 5 minutes).
      (3) Rectal (e.g., methohexital 10% 25 mg/kg acts within 7 minutes on average).
      (4) IV (e.g., thiopental, propofol, ketamine, midazolam). NB: younger infants are more sensitive to cardiorespiratory depressant effects of anesthetics.
      (5) Inhalation (e.g., halothane mask induction increased by 0.5% every 2 to 3 breaths; other volatile anesthetics tend to produce laryngospasm or coughing).
   b. Muscle Relaxation
      (1) Depolarizing agents: succinylcholine IV 2 mg/kg in neonates because of their increased body water composition; otherwise 1 mg/kg; IM 4 mg/kg
      (2) Nondepolarizing agents: atracurium 0.5 mg/kg or vecuronium 0.1 mg/kg
   c. Anticholinergic: IV atropine 0.02 mg/kg; maximum 0.6 mg often given on induction to prevent bradycardia induced by succinylcholine, halothane, and airway manipulation. Administration of IM atropine before surgery is ineffective.
   d. Example of typical anesthesia induction in healthy child:
      (1) Preoperative evaluation.
      (2) Rectal methohexital administered while child is in bed or in parent's arms.
      (3) Child is brought to OR asleep.
      (4) SaO_2 and precordial stethoscope placed.

(5) Sleep deepened by N_2O and halothane.
(6) ECG pads, BP cuff, and IV placed.
(7) Child is intubated without relaxant when anesthesia is deep enough.
(8) Bilateral breath sounds and air leak around ETT at 20 to 30 cm H_2O PIP confirmed.

SURGICAL PROCEDURE Appendectomy

Diagnosis of appendicitis may be difficult and delayed in children, increasing the risk of rupture.

Objective Removal of inflamed or perforated appendix; removal of abscess collections associated with appendicitis.

Position Supine.

Exposure Costal margin to groin.

Incision Right lower quadrant, transverse, or muscle splitting.

Nerves Involved The parietal peritoneum is innervated by the somatic segmental nerves T10 to L1. The visceral peritoneum, however, derives its nerve supply from higher sympathetic nerves. Thus a T4–6 block is required.

Blood Bank Order T&S or none.

Estimated Blood Loss Minimal.

Preoperative Studies CBC, electrolytes, BUN, creatinine, glucose.

Anesthetic Choices General or regional or both. General preferred. Regional is well tolerated but is relatively contraindicated in a septic patient.

Invasive Monitoring None.

Airway Considerations Routine.

Aspiration Precautions Yes.
1. H_2 blocker or gastrokinetic agent or both as premedications.
2. Since all these patients are considered to have full stomachs, either a rapid-sequence induction with cricoid pressure or an awake intubation should be used. Regional technique may be used as an alternative.

Estimated Surgical Time 30 to 60 minutes.

➤ **Anesthetic Considerations**
  1. **Preoperative Evaluation**
     Preoperative routine evaluation; and pay special attention to fluid and metabolic (Na, Cl, glucose) status of patient. Preoperative optimi-

zation without delaying procedure too much. Perioperative antibiotics started.

2. **Anesthetic Management**
   a. *Induction:* Rapid sequence.
   b. *Maintenance:* Fluids increased 7% to 10% for each degree Celsius of temperature elevation. Relaxation useful for surgical exposure; however, beware of short duration of procedure.
   c. *Emergence:* Awake extubation.

Intraoperative Hazards
1. Rupture of appendix; bacteremia.
2. Hemorrhage from slipped ligature.

Postoperative Pain Intensity   Moderate.

Postoperative Pain Control   Single-shot caudal: bupivacaine 0.125% to 0.25% with epinephrine 0.75 to 1 ml/kg. Routine analgesics.

SURGICAL PROCEDURE   Brachial Cleft Cyst Excision

Defects in development of brachial arch system produce fistula or cyst in lateral aspect of neck. Mucus frequently drains onto neck, which becomes infected. Most often extends from nasopharynx (tonsillar pillar) through to the neck surface, anterior to sternocleidomastoid.

Objective   Removal of congenital remnant of second brachial cleft.

Position   Supine, head to side opposite lesion.

Exposure   Mouth to mastoid to clavicle below and across midline.

Incision   Overlying the exit site. Occasionally, second high cervical incision needed for complete excision.

Blood Bank Order   None.

Estimated Blood Loss   Minimal.

Preoperative Studies   Routine.

Anesthetic Choice   General with oral endotracheal tube (OETT).

Invasive Monitoring   None.

Airway Considerations   Routine.

Aspiration Precautions   None unless child is at risk of gastric reflux.

Estimated Surgical Time   60 minutes.

➤ **Anesthetic Considerations**
1. Routine pediatric considerations
2. Short procedure
3. Lack of access to head

Intraoperative Hazards
1. ETT displacement, kinking.
2. Stimulation of carotid body as tract is dissected between internal and external carotid arteries.

Postoperative Pain Intensity   Mild to moderate.

Postoperative Pain Control   Parenteral, oral analgesics.

Postoperative Tests   Routine.

SURGICAL PROCEDURE   Biliary Atresia: Exploration

1. Congenital obstruction of bile duct. Most common cause is intrinsic obstruction from biliary atresia with complete blockage of part or all of the biliary tree. Atresias may be intrahepatic or extrahepatic.
2. Results in obstructive jaundice and biliary cirrhosis.
3. Exploration performed most often in first or second month of life.

Objective   Identify extrahepatic ducts. If none is present, surgeon will proceed with a portoenterostomy (Kasai procedure).

Position   Supine.

Exposure   Nipples to groin.

Incision   Right subcostal transverse.

Blood Bank Order   T&C 4 pediatric units PRBCs and 1 unit fresh frozen plasma.

Estimated Blood Loss   May be extensive because of hepatic dysfunction (abnormal PT and PTT) and portal hypertension.

Preoperative Studies   HCT, electrolytes, BUN, creatinine, calcium, glucose, PT, PTT, platelets, LFTs, albumin, bilirubin, CXR.

Anesthetic Choices   General with endotracheal intubation. If no underlying coagulopathy, consider a combined technique (general and regional).

Invasive Monitoring   Arterial line, central venous catheter.

Airway Considerations   Routine.

Aspiration Precautions   Consider awake intubation or rapid-sequence induction in the patient with appreciable ascites.

Estimated Surgical Time   3 to 6 hours.

➤ **Anesthetic Considerations**
1. **Preoperative Evaluation**
   a. Associated anomalies (especially malrotation and situs inversus).
   b. Obstructive jaundice, coagulopathy, ascites, liver dysfunction.
2. **Anesthetic Management**
   a. Routine neonatal considerations.
   b. Bleeding tendency.
   c. Respiratory compromise due to ascites and intrapulmonary shunts.
   d. Whether to use awake intubation or rapid-sequence induction depends on how ill the child is.
   e. Maintain on oxygen, air or N_2O, halothane, and a relaxant.
   f. Postoperative ventilation is required for varying periods.

Intraoperative Hazards
1. Bleeding, especially with portal hypertension
2. Hypoxemia
3. Hepatorenal syndrome
4. Hypoglycemia
5. Allergic reactions to cholangiographic dye

Postoperative Management   Pediatric ICU.

Postoperative Problems
1. Prolonged drug effects.
2. Hypoglycemia.
3. Bleeding.
4. Third space losses.
5. Parenteral alimentation may be required.

Postoperative Pain Intensity   Moderate to severe.

Postoperative Pain Control   Parenteral narcotics. Use narcotics with caution in patient with severe hepatic dysfunction.

Postoperative Tests   HCT, electrolytes, BUN, creatinine, calcium, glucose, PT, PTT, platelets.

SURGICAL PROCEDURE   Bronchoscopy for Foreign Body or Peanut Aspiration

Objective   Removal of foreign body from tracheobronchial tree.

Position   Supine.

Blood Bank Order   None.

Estimated Blood Loss   None.

Preoperative Studies CBC, CXR.

Anesthetic Choice General.

Airway Considerations Routine.

Aspiration Precautions Yes unless done electively.

Estimated Surgical Time Less than 30 minutes.

➤ **Anesthetic Considerations**
1. **Anesthetic Problems**
   a. Full stomach.
   b. Possible respiratory distress, $\dot{V}/\dot{Q}$ mismatch, hypoxia, septic state from postobstructive pneumonia. Foreign body may not be visible on CXR. Inspiratory and expiratory films useful in localizing foreign body.
   c. Pediatric procedure.
   d. Positive pressure ventilation may drive foreign body deeper into tracheobronchial tree.
   e. Spontaneous ventilation, on the other hand, may decrease control of airway and risk patient movement at critical moments.
   f. Ventilation can be provided through side arm of rigid bronchoscope.
   g. In complete tracheal main stem obstruction from peanut, surgeon pushes nut distal with rigid bronchoscope to allow ventilation. It is then retrieved quickly.
2. **Anesthetic Techniques**
   a. For emergency procedure done with full stomach considerations, use rapid-sequence induction and intubate for airway protection. Endotracheal tube switched to rigid bronchoscope with cricoid pressure. Reintubate after bronchoscopy. Extubate awake.
   b. If patient is not experiencing respiratory distress, procedure may be done semielectively, thus without aspiration precautions and without intubation. Anesthesia is induced and maintained with inhalation anesthesia and spontaneous ventilation. Induction may be slower than expected because of $\dot{V}/\dot{Q}$ mismatch.

Intraoperative Hazards
1. Patient's movement
2. Intraoperative desaturation
3. Aspiration while airway is unprotected
4. Occlusion of glottis by foreign body
5. Possible arrhythmias
6. Bronchospasm
7. Tooth damage

Postoperative Problems
1. Atelectasis
2. Pneumothorax

Postoperative Tests CXR.

SURGICAL PROCEDURE Circumcision

Objective Removal of excess foreskin. Correction of phimosis or paraphimosis.

Position Supine, frog-leg.

Exposure Suprapubic—perineum.

Incision Circumferential at glans penis.

Blood Bank Order None.

Estimated Blood Loss None.

Preoperative Studies Routine.

Anesthetic Choices General, regional, or local.
1. General: mask anesthetic.
2. Regional: caudal, epidural, or penile block.

Invasive Monitoring None.

Airway Considerations Routine.

Aspiration Precautions None unless child is at risk of gastric reflux.

Estimated Surgical Time Less than 30 minutes.

➤ **Anesthetic Considerations**
1. Routine pediatric considerations
2. Short procedure

Postoperative Pain Intensity Mild to moderate.

Postoperative Pain Control Oral analgesics; penile block. Penile block routinely performed at the completion of the procedure: provides 6 to 8 hours of postoperative analgesia.

Postoperative Tests None.

SURGICAL PROCEDURE Cleft Lip and Palate Repair

Common: 1.5 in 1000 live births; 25% of cases have isolated cleft lip; 50% have combination cleft lip and palate; 25% have isolated cleft palate. Cleft lip repair typically performed in infant 1 to 3 months of age; cleft palate at 1 to 2 years.

Objective Closure of clefts, permitting separation of oral and nasal cavities.

Repair important for speech development, decreased incidence of ear infection, and allowance for normal growth of maxilla.

Position   Supine with head extended.

Exposure   Full face.

Incision   Lip incisions for cleft lip; intraoral incisions for cleft palate.

Preoperative Studies   Routine.

Blood Bank Order   T&C 1 unit PRBCs for palate repair.

Estimated Blood Loss   Usually minimal with cleft lip repair, but blood loss appreciable in cleft palate repairs. Hold 1 unit PRBCs available.

Anesthetic Choice   General.

Invasive Monitoring   None.

Airway Considerations
1. Associated with Pierre Robin syndrome (brachygnathia and cleft palate); makes sucking and swallowing difficult; aspiration is common. Also associated with Treacher Collins syndrome (mandibulofacial dysostosis).
2. Endotracheal tube (ETT) considerations. Accidental extubation common.

Aspiration Precautions   Routine on induction, but full aspiration precautions on emergence (blood in stomach).

Estimated Surgical Time   Varies from 2 to 10 hours. Procedure often done in stages.

➤ **Anesthetic Considerations**
1. **Preoperative Evaluation**
   Associated anomalies in >10% of cases. Also significant association with airway abnormalities, namely Pierre Robin and Treacher Collins syndromes.
2. **Anesthetic Management**
   a. Antisialogogue (atropine 0.02 mg/kg IV) on induction.
   b. Conventional inhalation induction after airway inspected.
   c. Orotracheal intubation with a preformed tube (RAE tube) sewed midline to lower lip, avoiding distortion of upper lip. Use mouth gag and pharyngeal pack for cleft palate. Constantly check for ETT kinking, extubation, and endobronchial intubation after head movement.
   d. Protect eyes.
   e. Epinephrine subcutaneous injection limited to 1 ml/kg of 1:200,000 (5 μg/kg).
   f. Ensure removal of pharyngeal pack: aspirate stomach before extubation.
   g. Avoid mask or other airway manipulation. Awake extubation (as opposed to deep extubation). Tongue stitch helps maintain patent airway after extubation and stimulates ventilation.

Intraoperative Hazards
1. Difficult intubation
2. Displacement of ETT
3. Accidental extubation or endobronchial intubation
4. Bleeding

Postoperative Problem   Difficulty feeding infant.

Postoperative Pain Intensity   Moderate.

Postoperative Pain Control   Parenteral narcotics; intraoperative local infiltrate helps initially.

SURGICAL PROCEDURE Epiglottitis Management

Objective   Secure airway.

Position   Sitting up, initially; patient is most comfortable in that position.

Blood Bank Order   None.

Estimated Blood Loss   None.

Preoperative Studies   None (except neck x-rays occasionally; see Anesthetic Considerations).

Anesthetic Choice   General.

Invasive Monitoring   None.

Airway Considerations   Definite difficult airway. See Anesthetic Considerations.

Aspiration Precautions   Yes.

➤ **Anesthetic Considerations**
  1. **Preoperative Evaluation**
      a. Assess airway, breathing, circulation without disturbing or exciting child. Do *not* start IV, examine throat of child, or draw blood tests.
      b. Consider cause of upper airway obstruction: foreign body, infection (e.g., epiglottitis, retropharyngeal abscess, peritonsilar abscess, croup), trauma, tumor, anatomic abnormalities.
      c. If child is stable and in no distress, lateral x-rays of soft tissues of neck are optional. Accompany child to imaging department.
      d. Stay with distressed child; accompany him yourself to OR. Keep him undisturbed and sitting up. Keep parents with him all the way through induction.
      e. Keep cricothyrotomy tray available; surgeon is standing by.
      f. Considerations for induction are

  (1) Difficult airway
  (2) Airway at risk for complete obstruction
  (3) Full stomach (though essentially ignored during induction)
  (4) Toxic child
 2. Anesthetic Management
   a. *Induction:* In OR, place SaO_2 monitor and precordial stethoscope. Induce anesthesia in sitting-up child with 100% oxygen and halothane. Have cricothyrotomy or transtracheal ventilation set available.
   b. *Maintenance:* When child loses consciousness, lay him back and deepen induction with gentle positive pressure. Place IV. Orally intubate with ETT one size smaller than ordinarily used for age while maintaining spontaneous ventilation. Immediately try to change tube to nasotracheal intubation for greater stability. Obtain laryngeal swab cultures. Secure ETT well. Keep child well sedated. Treat with ampicillin, chloramphenicol, or cephalosporin (second or third generation antibiotic) to cover *Haemophilus influenzae* type B.

Postoperative Management   Monitor in ICU. Patients often left to breathe spontaneously in ICU. Will require good sedation and restraints to avoid self-extubation. Consider extubation 2 days later, when leak occurs around ETT.

Intraoperative Hazards   Complete respiratory obstruction. May press on chest to identify vocal cords (as air bubbles leak out) and attempt oral endotracheal intubation. Otherwise, immediately resort to surgical airway.

Postoperative Problems   Accidental or self-extubation because of agitation. Accidental extubation may be fatal.

Postoperative Tests   CXR, CBC, electrolytes, glucose, blood cultures, pharyngeal swabs.

SURGICAL PROCEDURE   Hirschsprung's Disease: Rectal Pull-through

Deficiency of ganglion cells, myenteric plexus of rectum, distal colon: causes chronic functional obstruction. Chronic constipation chief presenting complaint. *Definitive treatment:* excision of the aganglionic segment of bowel by abdominoperineal pull-through.

Objective   Removal and bypass of aganglionic distal colon to relieve constipation.

Position   Supine, with or without a simultaneous lithotomy position for exposure.

Exposure   Nipples to midthigh circumferentially.

Incision   Paramedian.

Blood Bank Order   T&C 2 pediatric units PRBCs.

Preoperative Studies   HCT, electrolytes, BUN, creatinine, glucose.

Anesthetic Choices   General with endotracheal intubations; or combined (general-regional) technique.

Invasive Monitoring   None.

Airway Considerations   Routine.

Aspiration Precautions   None unless patient is at risk of gastric reflux.

Estimated Surgical Time   2 to 4 hours.

➤ **Anesthetic Considerations**
   1. Routine pediatric considerations.
   2. Appreciable third space losses and fluid requirements.

Intraoperative Hazards   Vagal stimulation from traction on the peritoneum.

Postoperative Management   Recovery room.

Postoperative Problems   Continued third space losses.

Postoperative Pain Intensity   Moderate to severe.

Postoperative Pain Control   Parenteral analgesics, continued epidural.

Postoperative Tests   Electrolytes, HCT, glucose.

SURGICAL PROCEDURE   Hypospadias Repair: Distal and Midshaft

Urethra terminates proximal to tip of penis. The orifice may be at any point on the shaft of the penis or in the perineum.

Objective   Straighten penis; construct neourethra to bring meatus to tip of penis.

Position   Supine; frog-leg position with folded towel under buttocks.

Exposure   Umbilicus to midthigh to perineum.

Incision   Circumcoronal with excision of chordee scar tissue on base. Neo-urethra created from ventral shaft skin turned upward from the dorsal foreskin tubularized as a free graft.

Nerves Involved   S2,3,4 (pudendal nerves) give rise to a dorsal nerve of the penis via the pudendal nerve. Parasympathetic innervation (vasodilator fibers to the erectile tissue of the penis) from the anterior rami of S2,3,4.

Blood Bank Order   None.

Estimated Blood Loss   50 to 100 ml.

Preoperative Study   HCT.

Anesthetic Choices   General; or combined general and epidural.

Invasive Monitoring   None.

Airway Considerations   Routine.

Aspiration Precautions   No.

Estimated Surgical Time   1 to 2 hours.

➤ **Anesthetic Considerations**
Routine pediatric considerations.

Postoperative Problems   Patient's removing foam dressing.

Postoperative Pain Intensity   Moderate.

Postoperative Pain Control   Parenteral narcotics, continuous epidural, single-shot caudal followed by parenteral narcotics. Single-shot caudal easily performed in young child. Child placed in lateral position at end of procedure while still asleep. Caudal performed with bupivacaine 0.25%, 0.5 ml/kg. Child awakened and extubated.

Postoperative Tests   Hematocrit.

SURGICAL PROCEDURE   Meckel's Diverticulum: Resection

---

1. Diverticulum persists in 1% to 2% of the general population.
2. It is found on terminal ileum, within 60 cm of appendix.
3. Lining may contain ectopic gastric mucosa, pancreatic tissue: causes peptic ulceration and painless bleeding. Diverticulum may also present as acute abdomen from perforation or as small-bowel obstruction due to intussusception.

Objective   Removal of congenital remnant of omphalomesenteric duct.

Position   Supine.

Exposure   Nipples to groin.

Incision   Right lower quadrant, transverse.

Blood Bank Order   T&C 2 pediatric units PRBCs.

Estimated Blood Loss   Preoperatively may be appreciable. Painless rectal bleeding is brisk and common. Rarely exsanguinating.

Preoperative Study   HCT.

Anesthetic Choices   General; regional optional.

Invasive Monitoring   None.

Airway Considerations   Routine.

Aspiration Precautions   If the patient presents with an acute abdomen or for emergency procedure.

Estimated Surgical Time   30 to 60 minutes.

➤ **Anesthetic Considerations**
Routine plus overall hemodynamic assessment (hypovolemic or bacteremic) and optimization; see General Pediatric Considerations.

Intraoperative Hazards   Vagal reflex from traction on the peritoneum.

Postoperative Management   Recovery room.

Postoperative Pain Intensity   Moderate to severe.

Postoperative Pain Control   Parenteral narcotics. Continuous epidural. Single-shot caudal followed by parenteral narcotics.

SURGICAL PROCEDURE   Neuroblastoma (Posterior Mediastinal Mass): Thoracic

Common malignant neoplasm in children. Occurs anywhere along sympathetic chain, often in first 5 years of life.

Objective   Excision of mass and any enlarged lymph node.

Position   Lateral decubitus (Fig. 2) or supine.

Exposure   Midline front and back; neck to abdomen.

Incision   Posterolateral thoracotomy or midline abdominal.

Nerves Involved   T2 to T8.

Blood Bank Order   T&C 2 units PRBCs.

Estimated Blood Loss   Moderate. May be massive.

Preoperative Studies   HCT, coagulation profile, electrolytes, glucose, calcium, BUN, creatinine, CXR.

Anesthetic Choices   General with endotracheal intubation (ETI); or general with ETI combined with lumbar or thoracic epidural.

Invasive Monitoring   Arterial line.

Airway Considerations   Respiratory compromise due to pulmonary compression: usually not due to tracheal involvement as in anterior mediastinal masses.

Aspiration Precautions   None unless risk of gastric reflux.

Estimated Surgical Time   4 to 6 hours.

➤ **Anesthetic Considerations**
1. Preoperative assessment: Pay special attention to pediatric age or size; radiation therapy and chemotherapy; tumor spread (e.g., pancytopenia due to marrow invasion); respiratory symptoms (due to lung compression).
2. Potential for massive blood loss.
3. May secrete neuroendocrine hormones (vasoactive intestinal polypeptide [VIP], catecholamines), elevating BP and depleting intravascular volume.
4. Anesthetic managed according to patient's age and exact tumor location. Although tumors may secrete catechols, it usually is unnecessary to give adrenergic blocking agents. Tumor manipulation may result in BP rise or arrhythmias.

Postoperative Management   Pediatric ICU.

Postoperative Pain Intensity   Severe.

Postoperative Pain Control   Parenteral narcotics, continuous epidural, intercostal nerve block, interpleural catheter.

Postoperative Tests   HCT, electrolytes, CXR, close monitoring of BP and intravascular volume status (i.e., urine output); coagulation profile optional.

SURGICAL PROCEDURE   Pyloromyotomy (Ramstedt Procedure)

Hypertrophic pyloric stenosis occurs in as many as 1 in 300 live births. Symptoms are projectile vomiting, dehydration, and hypochloremic alkalosis. Vomit does not contain bile; vomiting occurs shortly after feeding.

Objective   Splitting hypertrophic muscle fibers of pylorus to relieve gastric outlet obstruction. Nitric oxide a likely initiator of pyloric stenosis.

Position   Supine.

Exposure   Nipples to groin.

Incision   Right-upper-quadrant transverse or right-subcostal-muscle splitting.

Blood Bank Order   None.

Estimated Blood Loss   Minimal.

Preoperative Studies   HCT, electrolytes, creatinine, BUN, ABGs, glucose.

Anesthetic Choice   General.

Invasive Monitoring   None.

Airway Considerations   Routine.

Aspiration Precautions   Yes. Aspirate stomach before induction.

Estimated Surgical Time   30 minutes.

➤ **Anesthetic Considerations**
1. **Preoperative Evaluation**
   Routine evaluation plus special attention to hydration state and metabolic abnormalities, namely, chloride, potassium, and acid-base balance. Acidosis implies severe dehydration.
2. **Optimization**
   Pyloromyotomy not an emergency procedure. Resuscitation and optimization essential before anesthetic. Preoperative nasogastric tube placement. Urine output is monitored.
3. **Anesthetic Management**
   Ensure adequate IV and routine monitoring.
   a. *Induction.* Intubate awake child or after rapid-sequence induction.
   b. *Maintenance.* Ensure good relaxation and control ventilation.
   c. *Emergence.* Extubate awake.

Postoperative Problems   Routine.

Postoperative Pain Intensity   Mild.

Postoperative Pain Control   Local infiltration with 0.5% bupivacaine, oral analgesics, IM narcotics.

SURGICAL PROCEDURE   Radiologic Procedures
_____

Includes magnetic resonance imaging (MRI), CT scans, and radiotherapy: Noninvasive high-resolution techniques. MRI provides excellent anatomic evaluation, superior to that of CT scan. No exposure to ionizing radiation.

Objectives   Diagnosis or therapy or both.

Preoperative Studies   Routine. Should be the same as for any other minor anesthetic.

Anesthetic Choices

1. General anesthesia. May involve endotracheal intubation (ETI) or spontaneous ventilation without ETI.
2. Monitored anesthesia care. Implies light IV or IM sedation so that patient is responsive to verbal stimulus.

➤ Anesthetic Considerations

1. **Requirements Related to Procedure**
   a. Common features
      (1) Radiologic suite remote from main anesthesia—OR.
      (2) Help less readily available.
      (3) Radiology personnel unfamiliar with anesthetic procedures.
      (4) Equipment problems (poor availability of suction, anesthetic equipment, resuscitation equipment).
      (5) Lack of access to patient and airway.
      (6) Claustrophobia when patient is in scanner. Closing eyes usually suppresses claustrophobia.
      (7) Requires immobility. Cooperation or general anesthetic required.
      (8) Room cold.
      (9) IV contrast medium. Severe reactions to it in 1% to 2% of patients. Those at risk have a history of atopic disease; allergy to seafood, shellfish, iodine; previous reactions to contrast media. Either do not expose or ensure prophylaxis with prednisone and diphenhydramine.
   b. CT scan: ionizing radiation exposure. Anesthetist far from patient.
   c. MRI. Specific to MRI is the magnetic field, which creates three major problems:
      (1) Ferromagnetic objects can be hurled toward the scanner.
      (2) Metallic objects, even nonferromagnetic ones, can degrade the image.
      (3) Electronic instruments and monitoring devices may not function properly within the vicinity of the magnet. Ferromagnetic objects: gas tanks, ventilators, laryngoscope batteries, stethoscopes, scissors, IV poles, wheelchairs, butterfly needles, pacemakers. Test by holding object tightly and slowly approaching magnet. Instruments not interfering with MRI: $ETCO_2$, noninvasive BP cuff, precordial plastic or aluminum stethoscope. Contraindications to MRI: aneurysm clips and pacemakers. Most heart valves not a problem.
2. **Requirements Related to Patient**
   Indications for general anesthesia: Young child, agitated or uncooperative adult, patient with movement disorder, patient requiring hyperventilation for elevated intracranial pressure.
3. **Requirements Related to Anesthesia**
   a. *Monitoring.* Most important is having the anesthesiologist able to monitor the patient closely by direct vision or by closed circuit TV. MRI requirements:
      (1) BP cuff, tubing, no metal connectors, automatic BP devices are used successfully.
      (2) ECG by telemetry or insulated wires.
      (3) Plastic precordial or esophageal stethoscope.
      (4) Capnography—long tubing with high suction.
      (5) Anesthesia machine is secured to wall far from magnet or special MRI-compatible machine.

b. *Anesthetic technique.*
  (1) For painless procedure for young children (3 months to 5 years old), hypnosis, plus insertion of IV for maintenance without intubation is recommended:
    (a) *Rectal approach:* brevital (25 mg/kg); IV sedation optional (rectal brevital good for 2 to 3 hours on its own).
    (b) *IM approach:* ketamine (3 to 7 mg/kg) and glycopyrrolate (0.05 to 0.1 mg); promethazine and chlorpromazine "cocktail."
    (c) *Oral approach:* chloral hydrate 70 mg/kg or midazolam 0.5 to 1.0 mg in sweet syrup. Maintenance may be obtained with IV ketamine, midazolam, propofol, or thiopental.
    (d) *IV approach:* propofol infusion (children require higher dosage than adults do).
  (2) In young children undergoing a painful procedure (IV contrast media is painful on injection) or in patient whose immobility is absolutely required (e.g., some radiotherapy), conventional general anesthesia with intubation and positive pressure ventilation is recommended.

Intraoperative Hazards
1. IV contrast media–induced allergic reaction or seizures.
2. Projectiles in MRI room.
3. Anesthesia-induced respiratory depression complicated by difficult access to patient.

SURGICAL PROCEDURE   Ranula Excision

Objective   Removal of mucous cyst from the floor of the mouth.

Position   Supine, mouth open.

Exposure   Oral cavity.

Incision   Around mass on floor of mouth.

Blood Bank Order   None.

Estimated Blood Loss   None.

Preoperative Study   HCT.

Anesthetic Choice   General with endotracheal intubation (ETI).

Invasive Monitoring   None.

Airway Considerations   Sharing the airway with the surgeons.

Aspiration Precautions   Not for induction; however, because of the risk of aspiration of blood during the procedure, either a cuffed tube or a throat pack should be used.

Estimated Surgical Time   60 minutes.

➤ **Anesthetic Considerations**
1. Routine pediatric considerations.
2. ETI required because of shared airway and aspiration of blood.

Intraoperative Hazards
1. Kinking or displacement of endotracheal tube.
2. Aspiration of blood.

Postoperative Problem Swelling: airway compromise if the nasal passages obstructed.

Postoperative Pain Intensity Mild to moderate.

Postoperative Pain Control Infiltration with local anesthetic. Oral analgesics.

SURGICAL PROCEDURE Tongue Tie Release

━━

Short frenulum restricts tongue movement around buccal sulcus.

Objective Release of congenitally short frenulum.

Position Supine.

Exposure Oral cavity.

Incision In frenulum, under tongue.

Blood Bank Order None.

Estimated Blood Loss Minimal.

Preoperative Studies Routine.

Anesthetic Choices General; local.

Invasive Monitoring None.

Airway Considerations
1. Share with surgeon.
2. Usually do not intubate: short procedure.

Aspiration Precautions Routine; suction blood in pharynx during procedure.

Estimated Surgical Time 2 minutes.

➤ **Anesthetic Considerations**
1. Antisialogogue.
2. Short procedure.
3. Inhalation induction and maintenance while sharing airway.

Intraoperative Hazards
1. Aspiration of blood
2. Laryngospasm

Postoperative Problems Routine.

Postoperative Pain Intensity Mild.

Postoperative Pain Control Infiltration with local anesthetic. Oral analgesics.

Postoperative Tests None.

SURGICAL PROCEDURE Tonsillectomy, Adenoidectomy, and
Reoperation for Bleeding Tonsils

Indications related to obstruction and infection.

Objective Removal of lymphoid tissue.

Position Supine.

Estimated Blood Loss Minimal.

Preoperative Studies Routine.

Anesthetic Choice General.

Airway Considerations Evaluate for symptoms of obstruction (snoring when asleep).

Aspiration Precautions Aspiration precautions present on emergence because of ingestion of blood.

Estimated Surgical Time Less than 30 minutes.

➤ **Anesthetic Considerations**
 1. **Preoperative Evaluation**
   a. Evaluation of symptoms of obstruction and extent of obstruction on physical examination. Avoid sedative premedication if obstruction severe.
   b. Evaluate for infection. Severe infection may necessitate deferring procedure until child is afebrile or free of upper respiratory tract infection, keeping in mind that some of these patients have frequent upper respiratory tract infections.
 2. **Anesthetic Technique**
   a. Antisialagogue useful.
   b. Consider awake intubation in patient with severe obstructive symptoms; potential for endotracheal tube (ETT) disconnection and dis-

placement; RAE tube useful; position ETT midline with bite block.
c. Remove pharyngeal packs at end of procedure.
d. Aspirate stomach and extubate child when awake because of certain ingestion of blood.

3. Reoperation for Bleeding

a. Intravascular volume depletion: Actual total bleeding difficult to evaluate. Orthostatic changes indicate 15% to 20% blood volume depletion. Always resuscitate child before reoperation. Keep large-bore IV and blood available. May consider ketamine induction.
b. Full stomach considerations: Requires rapid-sequence induction or awake intubation because of ingestion of large amounts of blood. Aspirate stomach after reoperation.
c. Anxious and irritable child.
d. See step 2 above for technique (i.e., antisialagogue, tube type, midline placement, etc.).

Intraoperative Hazards
1. Airway obstruction on induction
2. ETT displacement or disconnection

Postoperative Problems
1. Bleeding
2. Nausea
3. Vomiting

Postoperative Pain Intensity   Moderate.

Postoperative Pain Control   Parenteral narcotics.

Postoperative Tests   HCT if significant or persistent postoperative bleeding.

Neonatal Procedures

GENERAL NEONATAL CONSIDERATIONS

It is important that the General Pediatric Considerations listed at the beginning of this chapter be adhered to in neonates, less so in older children. Additional considerations for neonates:
1. Always consider associated congenital abnormalities.
2. Apnea of prematurity in infant with gestational age <44 weeks: postoperative monitoring in NICU for 24 hours.
3. Retinopathy of prematurity is a concern for neonates <44 weeks. Maintain SaO_2 at 90% to 95% or PaO_2 at 50 to 70 mm Hg.
4. Transitional circulation: reversal to fetal pattern of circulation may occur if neonate is hypoxic or acidotic. Reversal exacerbates hypoxia and introduces risk of paradoxical air embolism.
5. Has greater sensitivity to cardiovascular and respiratory depression from anesthetics.
6. Use of N_2O contraindicated (needs air; 100% oxygen optional) in congenital lobar emphysema, bronchial cyst, closed air space, and GI obstructions (volvulus, congenital diaphragmatic hernia, epiglottitis).
7. Special equipment: all warming measures, pediatric breathing circuit, IV Buretrol or infusion pump, intubation equipment; drugs drawn mostly in tuberculin syringes. Think small!
8. Arterial-line monitoring on right side—preductal.
9. Intubation technique: often awake if child is sick.

SURGICAL PROCEDURE   Congenital Lobar Emphysema: Lobectomy

One lobe involved usually, often left upper lobe. Coexistent congenital heart disease in 10% of cases. Progressive respiratory distress with unilateral thoracic hyperexpansion and atelectasis of contralateral lung. Increasing respiratory and cardiovascular compromise.

Objective   Resection of emphysematous lung tissue.

Position   Lateral decubitus.

Exposure   Midline front and back, neck to abdomen.

Incision   Thoracotomy of involved side.

Blood Bank Order   T&C 2 to 4 pediatric units PRBCs.

Estimated Blood Loss   100 to 400 ml.

Preoperative Studies   ABGs, HCT, electrolytes, BUN, creatinine, glucose, PT, PTT, platelets, CXR.

Anesthetic Choice   General with endotracheal intubation.

Invasive Monitoring   Right-sided arterial line (preductal).

Airway Considerations   If ventilation is required, maintain lowest peak positive airway pressures.

Aspiration Precautions   No.

Estimated Surgical Time   2 to 3 hours.

➤ **Anesthetic Considerations**
 1. **Preoperative Evaluation**
    Evaluation of respiratory compromise, associated anomalies.
 2. **Anesthetic Problems**
    a. Respiratory and cardiovascular compromise with increasing intrathoracic pressures.
    b. Positive pressure ventilation expands lobe by ball-valve effect.
    c. Spontaneous ventilation recommended until chest is open.
    d. N$_2$O contraindicated: prevents expansion of emphysematous lobe.
    e. Emergent decompression with chest tube used to relieve elevated intrathoracic pressures, although large leak is created.
    f. Neonatal considerations.
 3. **Anesthetic Management**
    a. Awake intubation.
    b. Spontaneous ventilation.
    c. Controlled ventilation with relaxation only after chest is opened.
    d. 100% oxygen or air and oxygen if patient can tolerate it.
    e. Extubation is planned for end of procedure.

Postoperative Management   NICU.

Postoperative Problem   Pneumothorax.

Postoperative Pain Intensity   Moderate to severe.

Postoperative Pain Control   Parenteral narcotics, continuous epidural.

Postoperative Tests   ABGs, electrolytes, HCT, glucose, CXR.

SURGICAL PROCEDURE   Diaphragmatic Hernia Repair

Most are present shortly after birth with respiratory distress. Mortality is high. Extracorporeal membrane oxygenator (ECMO) is sometimes indicated.
    Most common diaphragmatic hernia is on posterolateral left side. There is respiratory distress at birth and a scaphoid abdomen. Bowel sounds are heard over the left side. Pulmonary hypoplasia is on affected side and in opposite lung. There are associated anomalies in 25% of cases.

Objective   Return of abdominal viscera to the abdominal cavity.

Position   Lateral decubitus.

Exposure   Clavicle to groin, front and back.

Incision   Abdominal (subcostal) approach is used most often; transthoracic sometimes used.

Blood Bank Order   T&C 2 pediatric units PRBCs.

Estimated Blood Loss   100 to 200 ml.

Preoperative Studies   HCT, electrolytes, creatinine, glucose, BUN, PT, PTT, platelets, ABGs, CXR. ABGs may reflect severe hypoxemia, hypercapnia, and acidosis. Hypercapnia not responsive to vigorous hyperventilation has high mortality.

Anesthetic Choice   General.

Invasive Monitoring   Arterial line; central venous catheter optional. Do not delay surgery to place an arterial line. After decompression, right radial artery line aids postoperative management. Arterial line placed on right side for assay of gases proximal to ductus arteriosus.

Airway Considerations   Avoid positive pressure mask ventilation (may further increase respiratory compromise by gastric distension). Awake intubation recommended.

Aspiration Precautions   No.

➤ **Anesthetic Considerations**
1. **Preoperative Evaluation**
   Routine neonatal evaluation, with special attention to associated anomalies and pulmonary compromise.
2. **Anesthetic Problems**
   a. Neonate.
   b. Associated anomalies.
   c. Often very ill neonate.
   d. Severe pulmonary compromise.
   e. Risk of pneumothorax higher on contralateral side.
   f. Persistent fetal or transitional circulation.
3. **Anesthetic Management**
   a. Preinduction
      (1) Decompress stomach with nasogastric tube (NGT).
      (2) Nurse the child in semiupright position.
      (3) Supplemental humidified oxygen or intubate.
   b. Intraoperative awake intubation: Avoid high airway pressures because of risk of pneumothorax. Use rapid, small tidal volumes. Avoid N_2O; 100% oxygen generally required. Muscle relaxation and postoperative ventilation required.

Postoperative Problem
1. Persistent fetal circulation (PFC): shunting across the foramen ovale and ductus arteriosus due to increased pulmonary vascular resistance (PVR).

Therefore avoid acidosis, hypothermia, hypoxemia, hypercapnia, elevated airway pressures, and noxious stimuli. Paralysis and continuous infusion of fentanyl may help decrease airway pressures and noxious stimuli.

2. Pneumothorax; acute decompensation mandates consideration of pneumothorax on contralateral side.

Postoperative Pain Intensity   Moderate to severe.

Postoperative Pain Control   Epidural, parenteral, continuous fentanyl infusion.

Postoperative Tests   HCT, electrolytes, creatinine, ABGs, BUN, glucose, calcium, CXR.

SURGICAL PROCEDURE   Esophageal Atresia with Tracheoesophageal Fistula (TEF) Repair

Most common form is esophageal atresia with fistula between distal esophagus and trachea. Usually detected when neonate chokes on first feed. Associated anomalies common, namely, VATER (Vertebral abnormalities, imperforate Anus, Tracheo-Esophageal fistula, Radial aplasia or Renal abnormalities) syndrome; 25% of patients also have cardiac anomalies. High incidence of prematurity.

Objective   Interruption of communication between trachea and esophagus, with primary anastomosis of esophagus.

Position   Lateral decubitus on side opposite aortic arch (usually right). A gastrostomy tube is often placed prior to the thoracic procedure.

Exposure   Lateral neck and arm along with lateral thorax to abdomen and midline anterior and posterior.

Incision   Lateral thoracotomy through T3–4 interspace. Occasionally, a second thoracotomy is done through a lower interspace. A second, cervical incision is made. If fistula is an H type, cervical approach is used primarily.

Blood Bank Order   T&C 2 pediatric units PRBCs.

Estimated Blood Loss   100 to 300 ml.

Preoperative Studies   HCT, electrolytes, BUN, creatinine, glucose, calcium, CXR; echocardiogram if suspect associated cardiac anomaly.

Anesthetic Choices   General with endotracheal intubation (ETI) or combined technique of general with ETI and a caudal catheter.

Invasive Monitoring   Right-sided arterial line (preductal), Foley catheter; central venous catheter optional. Arterial line useful to monitor blood gases.

Airway Considerations   Communication between esophagus and trachea causes gastric distension during positive pressure ventilation that subsequently further compromises ventilation. Endotracheal tube (ETT) should be positioned immediately distal to the fistula. This can be accomplished by intubating the right main stem and then slowly withdrawing the ETT until bilateral breath sounds are heard.

With type-1 TEF (no communication between esophagus and trachea), use routine induction. Otherwise, perform awake intubation while maintaining spontaneous ventilation until chest is open.

Aspiration Precautions   Patient is at risk for pulmonary aspiration until fistula is ligated.

Estimated Surgical Time   2 hours.

Queries for Surgeon   Staged procedures or primary repair.

Estimated Surgical Time   2 hours.

➤ **Anesthetic Considerations**
  1. **Preoperative Evaluation and Optimization**
     a. Routine evaluation. Pay special attention to associated anomalies (VATER and cardiac) and to pulmonary status because of the high risk of aspiration pneumonitis.
     b. NPO.
     c. Soft rubber tube to decompress esophageal pouch.
     d. Upright posture to prevent regurgitation.
     e. Gastrostomy preinduction optional.
  2. **Anesthetic Problems**
     a. Sick premature infant or neonate.
     b. Associated anomalies.
     c. Pulmonary compromise due to aspiration.
     d. Positive pressure ventilation (PPV) without a gastrostomy may distend stomach, further compromising respiration.
  3. **Anesthetic Management**
     a. Awake intubation maintaining spontaneous ventilation.
     b. When PPV required, avoid N_2O. Either place gastrostomy or avoid vigorous positive pressure. Wait until fistula is ligated, or place tip of ETT below fistula.
     c. When chest is open, give relaxant and control ventilation.
     d. Attempt early postoperative extubation to avoid stress on tracheal sutures. Prolonged respiratory care may be required.

Postoperative Management   NICU.

Postoperative Problem   Tracheomalacia or recurrent laryngeal nerve injury may cause airway obstruction postoperatively.

Postoperative Pain Intensity   Moderate to severe.

Postoperative Pain Control   Parenteral narcotics, continuous epidural.

SURGICAL PROCEDURE Gastroschisis Repair

Herniation of abdominal contents through a full-thickness defect in abdominal wall lateral to umbilicus, which is situated normally. Bowel is exposed to external environment. Associated congenital defects rare. Incidence is 1 in 15,000 live births.

Objective Return bowel to abdominal cavity. May require a staged procedure using a prosthetic silo.

Position Supine.

Exposure Nipples to groin.

Incision Around abdominal wall defect.

Blood Bank Order T&C 2 pediatric units PRBCs.

Estimated Blood Loss 100 to 200 ml.

Preoperative Studies HCT, electrolytes, creatinine, BUN, glucose, calcium, ABGs, PT, PTT, platelets, CXR.

Anesthetic Choices General with endotracheal intubation.

Invasive Monitoring Foley, arterial line.

Airway Considerations Routine.

Aspiration Precautions Yes.

Estimated Surgical Time 2 to 3 hours.

➤ **Anesthetic Considerations**
1. **Preoperative Evaluation**
   Pay special attention to associated anomalies, third space losses, temperature instability, preoperative optimization.
2. **Anesthetic Problems**
   a. Premature infant or neonate (see General Neonatal Considerations).
   b. Extensive heat and fluid losses from herniated sac before and during surgery.
   c. Respiratory and cardiovascular compromise with replacement of bowel in abdominal cavity.
3. **Anesthetic Management**
   a. *Preoperative.* Evaluation, resuscitation. Cover extraabdominal bowel with moist gauze and plastic wrap. Nasogastric tube used to decompress bowel. Conventional setup for neonate.
   b. *Intraoperative.* Intubation usually performed in awake neonate because of his degree of illness. Avoid N_2O to help prevent bowel distension. Relaxation is required to facilitate replacement of bowel in abdominal cavity. Postoperative controlled ventilation frequently required.

Postoperative Management   NICU.

Postoperative Problems   Large third space losses. Because of encroachment of abdominal contents on diaphragm, postoperative ventilatory support required.

Postoperative Pain Intensity   Moderate to severe.

Postoperative Pain Control   Parenteral narcotics, continuous epidural.

Postoperative Tests   HCT, electrolytes, creatinine, BUN, glucose, ABGs, CXR.

SURGICAL PROCEDURE   Intestinal Surgery

Perineal Anoplasty   Surgical repair for imperforate anus. Normal anal opening absent: most often is associated with a fistula (e.g., rectoperineal or rectovaginal); 25% to 75% of patients have other associated congenital abnormalities; 10% has esophageal atresia without a tracheoesophageal fistula (TEF). VATER (Vertebral abnormalities, imperforate Anus, Tracheo-Esophageal fistula, Radial aplasia or Renal abnormalities) syndrome is associated. Bilateral renal agenesis is fatal.

Meconium Ileus   Invariably associated with cystic fibrosis. Intestinal obstruction occurs most often at level of the ileum because of incompletely digested meconium. Enterostomy may be necessary if conservative measures fail.

Intestinal Atresia   Complete obstruction because of mucosal diaphragm or interruption of continuity of bowel. Most common at duodenum and ileum. Associated with Down syndrome.

Duodenal Atresia   Diagnosis suggested by bilious vomiting soon after birth and "double bubble" sign on x-ray examination; 20% incidence of associated congenital anomalies, especially trisomy 21 (Down syndrome) and cardiac defects.

Malrotation and Midgut Volvulus   Incomplete rotation of the gut during embryonic life permits volvulus of the gut. Volvulus causes atretic segments, intestinal obstruction, and vascular compromise.

Objective   To relieve GI obstruction.

Position   Supine (Fig. 1), lithotomy (Fig. 3), or prone jackknife (Fig. 6).

Exposure   Abdominal; perineum optional.

Incision   Abdominal; circumanal optional.

Blood Bank Order   T&C 2 pediatric units PRBCs.

Estimated Blood Loss   Minimal to several hundred milliliters.

Preoperative Studies CBC, BUN, electrolytes, creatinine, glucose, calcium, PT, PTT, CXR.

Anesthetic Choices General with endotracheal intubation (ETI) or general with ETI combined with epidural.

Invasive Monitoring If child is very ill.

Airway Considerations Routine.

Aspiration Precautions Full stomach. Rapid-sequence induction or awake intubation.

Estimated Surgical Time 2 to 3 hours.

➤ **Anesthetic Considerations**
  1. **Preoperative Evaluation**
     a. Associated congenital abnormalities.
     b. Third-space requirements and hypothermia.
     c. Preoperative optimization of hemodynamic, fluid, and metabolic abnormalities.
     d. Neonatal considerations.
  2. **Anesthetic Management**
     a. Awake intubation or rapid-sequence induction.
     b. Conventional anesthetic with neonatal considerations.

Postoperative Management Pediatric ICU.

Postoperative Problems Routine.

Postoperative Pain Intensity Moderate.

Postoperative Pain Control Parenteral narcotics or continuous epidural or caudal.

Postoperative Tests CBC, electrolytes, creatinine, BUN, glucose.

SURGICAL PROCEDURE Necrotizing Enterocolitis: Exploration
_____

Potentially life-threatening neonatal condition; found especially in low-birth-weight infants.

Partial or generalized necrosis of mucosa; sometimes of submucosa of small or large bowel, or both. Associated with birth asphyxia, premature infants, respiratory distress syndrome, and shock.

Clinical picture: abdominal distension, temperature instability, bloody diarrhea, apnea, bradycardia spells. Definitive diagnosis is established by pneumatosis intestinalis on x-ray films.

Objective Remove compromised bowel and establish stoma or stomas. Drain abscess.

Position Supine.

Exposure Nipples to groin.

Incision Transverse or midline.

Blood Bank Order T&C 2 to 4 pediatric units of washed cells and 2 to 4 units of fresh frozen plasma (FFP). Platelets may be required. Use washed cells to avoid hemolysis caused by Thompson-Friedenrich cryptantigen (TFC) on RBC surfaces. FFP should also be screened for TFC.

Preoperative Studies Electrolytes, creatinine, BUN, HCT, PT, PTT, platelets, glucose, calcium, ABGs. Patients may have a metabolic acidosis secondary to sepsis. Thrombocytopenia is frequently present.

Anesthetic Choice General.

Invasive Monitoring Arterial line, central venous catheter, Foley.

Airway Considerations Controlled ventilation.

Aspiration Precautions Yes. Many patients will come to the OR intubated. If not, use either awake intubation or rapid-sequence induction with cricoid pressure. Awake intubation preferred.

Estimated Surgical Time Variable; depends on extent of resection.

➤ **Anesthetic Considerations**
 1. **Preoperative Evaluation**
     a. Critically ill neonate
     b. Extent of prematurity or low birth weight
     c. Associated anomalies
     d. Laboratory studies
 2. **Anesthetic Problems**
     a. Hemodynamic and fluid status
     b. Respiratory distress
     c. Metabolic abnormalities
     d. Coagulopathy
     e. Sepsis and antibiotic requirements
     f. Temperature instability
     g. Prematurity and neonatal issues
 3. **Anesthetic Management**
     Postoperative neonatal anesthetic considerations. Pay special attention to above issues. Postoperative ventilation.

Postoperative Management NICU.

Postoperative Pain Intensity Moderate.

Postoperative Pain Control Parenteral narcotics.

Postoperative Tests Electrolytes, creatinine, BUN, HCT, PT, PTT, platelets, glucose, calcium, ABGs.

SURGICAL PROCEDURE Omphalocele Closure

Compare with Gastroschisis Repair discussion. Omphalocele is the herniation of abdominal contents through the abdominal wall. Apex of sac is the umbilicus. Bowel is covered by a membranous sac. Associated congenital defects are more common with omphalocele (occur in approximately 75% of cases) than with gastroschisis. They include exstrophy of the bladder, congenital heart disease, and Beckwith-Wiedemann syndrome (associated with severe hypoglycemia). Ruptured omphalocele yields large third space losses.

Objective Reduction of abdominal contents from omphalocele and closure of the abdominal wall. The size of the defect and the organs involved determine whether the procedure needs to be done in stages.

Position Supine.

Exposure Nipples to groin.

Incision Around omphalocele.

Blood Bank Order T&C 2 pediatric units PRBCs.

Estimated Blood Loss 100 ml.

Preoperative Studies HCT, electrolytes, creatinine, BUN, PT, PTT, platelets, glucose, calcium, CXR.

Anesthetic Choice General with endotracheal intubation.

Invasive Monitoring Foley, arterial line.

Airway Considerations Pay special attention to associated congenital anomalies. Patients with Beckwith-Wiedemann syndrome have large tongues, predisposing them to airway difficulties.

Aspiration Precautions Yes. Awake intubation or rapid-sequence induction.

Estimated Surgical Time 2 to 3 hours.

➤ **Anesthetic Considerations**
See Gastroschisis Repair.

Postoperative Management NICU.

Postoperative Problems
1. Pneumothorax
2. Hypothermia
3. Fluid shifts
4. Compromise of venous return
5. Ventilatory support required
6. Total parenteral nutrition (TPN) required

Postoperative Pain Intensity   Moderate to severe.

Postoperative Pain Control   Parenteral narcotics, continuous epidural.

Postoperative Tests   HCT, electrolytes, creatinine, BUN, glucose, calcium, ABGs, CXR.

SURGICAL PROCEDURE   Patent Ductus Arteriosus (PDA) Ligation

There are two major presentations:
1. Premature neonate with associated respiratory distress syndrome, often complicated by congestive heart failure.
2. Older infant or young child with an asymptomatic murmur.
PDA produces left-to-right shunt. Magnitude determined by PDA size and ratio of systemic to pulmonary resistances. Large PDA causes congestive heart failure and pulmonary hypertension.

Objective   Relief of left-to-right shunt.

Position   Lateral decubitus.

Exposure   Midline front and back, neck to abdomen.

Incision   Lateral thoracotomy.

Blood Bank Order   T&C 2 pediatric units PRBCs.

Estimated Blood Loss   Minimal.

Preoperative Studies   HCT, electrolytes, BUN, creatinine, glucose, calcium, CXR, ECG, cardiac studies (echocardiogram, catheterization).

Anesthetic Choices   General with endotracheal intubation (ETI); general with ETI and epidural catheter.

Invasive Monitoring   Arterial line.

Airway Considerations   Routine.

Aspiration Precautions   None unless an emergency procedure or child is at risk of gastric reflux.

Estimated Surgical Time   30 to 60 minutes.

➤ **Anesthetic Considerations**
  1. Anesthetic Problems
      a. Associated severe respiratory compromise in premature infants due to respiratory distress syndrome or bronchopulmonary dysplasia.
      b. Precautions for premature neonate (see General Neonatal Considerations).

    c. Vagal nerve stimulation or injury may occur during dissection.
    d. Remove all air bubbles in IVs. Potential reversal of shunt would result in paradoxical air embolism.
    e. Do not decrease the systemic vascular resistance and increase the pulmonary vascular resistance to a point that reversal of the shunt occurs.

2. Anesthetic Management
    a. Standard neonatal anesthetic.
    b. Intubate awake with IV induction or inhalation induction, depending on status.

Intraoperative Hazards
1. Massive bleeding
2. Damage to recurrent laryngeal nerve
3. Compression of lung

Postoperative Management   NICU.

Postoperative Pain Intensity   Moderate to severe.

Postoperative Pain Control   Parenteral narcotics, continuous epidural, intercostal blocks.

SUGGESTED READINGS

Coté CJ, Ryan JF, Todres ID, Goudsouzian NG. A Practice of Anesthesia for Infants and Children, ed. 2. Philadelphia: W.B. Saunders, 1993.

Steward, D. Manual of Pediatric Anesthesia. New York: Churchill Livingstone, 1985.

Cook DR. Pediatric Anesthesia. In Barash P (Ed). Clinical Anesthesia. London: J.B. Lippincott, 1992.

CHAPTER 11

PLASTIC SURGERY PROCEDURES

GENERAL CONSIDERATIONS FOR RECONSTRUCTIVE PLASTIC SURGERY

This discussion covers common reconstructive operations that typically do not involve grafts or flaps. Includes reconstruction of facial soft tissues: brow lift, blepharoplasty, face lift; and breast augmentation, reconstruction, and reduction. Occasionally procedure involves cartilage or bone graft taken from distant site.

Objective   Provide aesthetic improvement of the face, neck, breasts, abdomen, and extremities.

Position   Depends on procedure and operative sites, but patient is almost always supine.

Exposure   Depends on operative site.

Incision   Depends on exact procedure.

Anesthetic Choices   General or local with IV sedation. Either anesthetic technique can be used in most facial aesthetic procedures. General can involve mask, laryngeal mask, or endotracheal tube.

Invasive Monitoring   Routine.

Airway Considerations   Facial procedures with complicated airway problems may require nasal, awake, or fiberoptic intubation.

Aspiration Precautions   Routine.

Queries for Surgeon   Expected duration of procedure so can tailor anesthetic time, since surgical speed quite variable?

➤ **Anesthetic Considerations**
   1. **Preoperative Considerations**
      a. Generally patient is healthy, although sometimes obese.
      b. Often done as outpatient procedure.
      c. Routine history, physical examination, and laboratory studies.

2. **Anesthetic Problems**
   a. Procedures may be very long, requiring special attention to positioning (possibility of compression injuries), and maintenance of body temperature.
   b. Vasoconstrictor soaks and an epinephrine-containing local anesthetic are frequently used.
   c. Procedures often are done with patient under local anesthesia (e.g., brow lift, facial aesthetic procedures).
   d. General anesthesia indicated in the following circumstances: patient preference, pediatric patients, claustrophobic patients, breast reduction procedures.
   e. Patient undergoing breast procedures are at risk for pneumothorax.
   f. Patients undergoing breast reduction may be difficult laryngoscopies because of large breasts. Short-handle laryngoscope is useful.
   g. Mask ventilation after the procedure is problematic in most facial procedures because of the risk of disturbing the repair.
   h. After prolonged procedures and procedures in which reintubation may be difficult, patient may benefit from a period of postoperative intubation and a slow wake-up, with extubation when fully awake.

Intraoperative Hazards
1. Local anesthesia toxicity
2. Inadvertent intravascular epinephrine administration
3. Accidental extubation in nonsupine position
4. Allergic reaction to any anesthetic or antibiotic
5. Position-related injuries

GENERAL CONSIDERATIONS FOR FLAPS AND GRAFTS

Includes anterior thigh, deltopectoral, gracilis, groin, latissimus dorsi, "pressure sore," and rectus abdominus flaps.

Objective   Mobilization of tissue to cover a soft tissue defect. A flap maintains the tissue blood supply intact; a graft depends on the recipient site's blood supply for nourishment. Thin skin grafts are 0.20 to 0.38 mm thick. Inadvertent movements of patient before the final dressing is applied may dislodge the graft. Plaster splints or casts are often used to maintain integrity of the graft. Polypropylene splints or casts applied by prosthetic technicians are better for patients and surgeon.

Position   Depends on procedure and operative sites.

Exposure   Depends on procedure and operative sites.

Incision   Depends on procedure and operative sites.

Blood Bank Order   Depends on procedure and operative sites.

Estimated Blood Loss   Can be considerable. Increased with multiple grafts, large areas of debridement, and with vascular and possibly microvascular anastomoses.

Preoperative Studies   Routine.

Anesthetic Choices   Regional or general. Distant locations of donor and recipient sites and long operative times are indications for general anesthesia.

Invasive Monitoring   Routine. Arterial line optional; Foley catheter for long procedures; and central venous catheter for long procedures with anticipated large fluid shifts and cardiac compromise.

Airway Considerations   Routine.

Aspiration Precautions   Routine.

Queries for Surgeon
1. Projected duration? (N.B.: Actual time may far exceed surgeon's projection.)
2. Estimated blood loss?

Estimated Surgical Time   Variable.

➤ **Anesthetic Considerations**
1. Prolonged procedures; some take >20 hours. Pay special attention to positioning to avoid compression injuries.
2. Closely monitor temperature and fluid status. Flaps are sensitive to hypoperfusion. Heparin or dextran 40 required to maintain blood flow in vessels to be joined. Administer dextran 1 (Promit) before dextran 40 to prevent allergic reaction. Blood and third space losses large because of extensive tissue dissection. Volume status aggressively maintained to avoid hypovolemia and the use of vasopressors.
3. Vasoconstrictor soaks and an epinephrine-containing local anesthetic are frequently used. In children under halothane anesthesia, limit epinephrine-containing solution (<5 μg/kg, i.e., 1 ml/kg of 1:200,000) to prevent arrhythmias.
4. *Emergence:* Narcotics required for relief of pain. Flaps and wounds closed under tension, so must be protected from injury caused by sudden patient movements or violent coughing. After prolonged procedures patients may have significant airway edema or blunted airway reflexes. May benefit from a short period of postoperative intubation and slow wake-up.

Intraoperative Hazards
1. Arrhythmias with vasoconstrictor with or without added local anesthesia
2. Concealed major blood loss
3. Hypothermia

Postoperative Management   PACU; occasionally ICU after very long procedures.

Postoperative Problems
1. Pain relief
2. Ischemia of flap
3. Continuing heparin or dextran to maintain adequate fluid volume and good hemodynamic status to optimize flap perfusion

4. Patient agitation, especially during transfer and emergence, resulting in flap or graft disruption

SURGICAL PROCEDURES Special Flaps

Anterior Thigh Flap Anterior thigh or groin defects; covering for exposed vascular prosthesis. **Position** supine. **Exposure** anterior thigh. **Incision** longitudinal anterior thigh.

Deltopectoral Flap Head and neck reconstruction. **Position** supine. **Exposure** upper hemithorax and shoulder. **Incision** oblique across upper chest to shoulder. A skin graft may be required to close the donor defect.

Gracilis Flap Perineal defects; vaginal reconstruction; donor for free tissue transfer **(free flap)**. **Position** supine and frog-legged. **Exposure** medial thigh or thighs. **Incision** directly over muscle.

Groin Flap Hand and forearm defects; local groin and abdominal wounds. **Position** supine with roll under hip. Down leg draped for mobility. **Exposure** wide groin and iliac crest. **Incision** oblique, parallel to the inguinal ligament.

Latissimus Dorsi Flap Chest wall, breast, head and neck, and upper arm reconstruction; donor for free tissue transfer **(free flap)**. **Position** lateral decubitus with arm draped so it can be moved. **Exposure** entire posterior hemithorax, anterior hemithorax, axilla, and upper arm. **Incision** anterior border of latissimus muscle.

"Pressure Sore" Flaps Gluteus maximus, biceps femoris, and posterior thigh flaps are used to cover defects over the sacrum, ischium, and buttock areas, most commonly due to pressure sores. **Position** prone. **Exposure** buttocks and posterior thigh. **Incision** all pressure sores are first debrided. Incisions are then made to move the chosen muscle into place. The gluteus flap for sacral closure is usually raised bilaterally through two medially based V incisions. The biceps femoris and posterior thigh muscles are approached through a long V incision on the back of the leg. **Anesthetic choices** general or regional.

Rectus Abdominis Flap With skin component: breast, chest wall, and groin reconstruction; without skin: chest wall, trunk, and sternal reconstruction; and as donor for free tissue transfer **(free flap)**. **Position** supine, flexion at waist can assist in relaxing the donor site for easy closure. **Exposure** wide abdominal. **Incision** with skin: surrounding skin paddle that overlies muscle or centered transversely above or below umbilicus. Without skin: paramedian incision.

SURGICAL PROCEDURE Abdominoplasty

Objective To improve abdominal contour by removing excess skin and fat and by tightening abdominal fascia. May be combined with liposuction and repair of diastasis recti abdominis.

Position Supine, with hip flexion to aid closure.

Exposure Abdomen, xiphoid to pubis.

Incision Wavy transverse, approximately in bikini swimsuit line.

Blood Bank Order T&S.

Estimated Blood Loss 100 to 500 ml.

Preoperative Studies Routine.

Anesthetic Choices General or regional.

Invasive Monitoring Not routine.

Airway Considerations May be difficult airway (mask and intubation) in obese patients.

Aspiration Precautions Use aspiration precautions for obese patients.

Estimated Surgical Time 2 hours.

➤ **Anesthetic Considerations**
1. Considerations for obese patients: Includes transport and positioning difficulties; difficulties with all techniques (IV, regional, endotracheal intubation); respiratory compromise accentuated by supine or Trendelenburg position; associated cardiovascular disease; and glucose intolerance.
2. Prevent coughing and struggling on emergence. Repair may dehisce. Consider extubation while patient is under deep anesthesia.
3. Fluid requirements dictated by blood loss and extent of liposuction (see Anesthetic Considerations for Liposuction below for fluid replacement).

Postoperative Pain Intensity Moderate.

Postoperative Pain Control Parenteral narcotics.

SURGICAL PROCEDURE Liposuction (Suction-assisted Lipectomy)

Objective Removal of excessive or maldistributed body fat.

Position Depends on location of fat to be removed. May require position changes to assess all locations.

Exposure Affected areas.

Incision   1 cm incisions in areas most accessible to suction cannulae.

Blood Bank Order   None or T&C 2 units PRBCs.

Estimated Blood Loss   Depends on extent of procedure.

Preoperative Studies   Routine.

Anesthetic Choices   General, regional, or local. Regional technique suitable for all liposuctions below costal margins. Tumescent liposuction (technique with prior subcutaneous administration of large volumes of dilute local anesthetic) done with patient under local anesthesia.

Invasive Monitoring   None.

Airway Considerations   Possible difficult airway in obese patients.

Aspiration Precautions   Yes if patient is obese.

➤ **Anesthetic Considerations**
1. **Considerations for Obese Patients**
   a. Technical difficulties (transport, positioning, IVs, epidural, intubation).
   b. Respiratory compromise (greater oxygen consumption, increased work of breathing, decreased functional residual capacity, $\dot{V}/\dot{Q}$ mismatch), cardiovascular disease (hypertension, coronary artery disease), GI reflux.
2. **Blood Loss**
   Removal of large amounts of fat requires appropriate fluid replacement. Fat removed by suction lipectomy is approximately 20% to 30% blood; additional blood loss into wound is highly variable. Men have much larger wound fluid losses and 3 times the blood loss of women. Removal of large fat volumes entails proportionate blood loss, as well as third space losses. The average crystalloid volume replacement is approximately 3 times the fat aspirate volume but needs to be individualized.
3. **Use of Local Anesthesia with Epinephrine**
   Lidocaine and epinephrine used for analgesia and hemostasis.

Postoperative Pain Intensity   Minimum to moderate.

Postoperative Pain Control   Oral narcotics.

SURGICAL PROCEDURE   Rhinoplasty or Septoplasty

Objective   Improvement of appearance of nose and of caliber of nasal airway.

Position   Supine with head elevated.

Exposure   Full face.

Incision   Intranasal.

Blood Bank Order   None.

Estimated Blood Loss   Less than 300 ml.

Preoperative Studies   Routine.

Anesthetic Choices   General with endotracheal intubation or local with sedation.

Invasive Monitoring   Not routine.

Airway Considerations   Endotracheal tube taped to mandible in midline. Pharyngeal packs used to collect blood and secretions.

Aspiration Precautions   Routine.

Estimated Surgical Time   1 hour.

➤ **Anesthetic Considerations**
1. Nose packed with topical vasoconstrictor (epinephrine) and lidocaine.
2. Pharyngeal pooling of blood and secretions; bleeding into posterior pharynx complicates airway management. Because the nose is obstructed with packing at extubation, pay special attention to maintaining a clear oropharynx.
3. Extubate fully awake: avoid mask ventilation after extubation as it may disturb rhinoplasty repair.

Postoperative Problems   Bleeding into pharynx; retained pharyngeal pack (disastrous).

Postoperative Pain Intensity   Minimum to moderate.

Postoperative Pain Control   Parenteral or oral.

SURGICAL PROCEDURE   Split-Thickness Skin Grafts for Burns

1. Skin defect may be due to a burn or such causes as pressure sores or ulcerations or a nonhealing wound or wound dehiscence, or skin defect may be created surgically by excision of a lesion or a flap or graft.
2. Burn patients can be very ill, depending on depth of burn, extent of burn, age of patient, and underlying medical problems.
3. Early excision and grafting in burns improves cosmetics and lessens morbidity and mortality.

Objective   Cover skin defect.

Position   Depends on procedure and operative sites.

Exposure   Depends on procedure and operative sites.

Incision   Depends on procedure and operative sites.

Blood Bank Order   T&C 2 units. Requires more if procedure is extensive.

Estimated Blood Loss   Depends on size and extent of debridement.

Preoperative Studies   CBC, coagulation profile, electrolytes, and as indicated.

Anesthetic Choices   General, regional, or local, depending on sites and extent of involvement. Bacteremia, hypovolemia, or involvement of back precludes regional anesthesia in patients with extensive burns.

Invasive Monitoring   Arterial line recommended for large burns.

Airway Considerations   Difficult airway may be short term (e.g., airway edema due to inhalation injury) or long term (e.g., neck and face scars limiting airway access). Extensive burns (>30% to 50% total body surface area) result in significant edema, including airway edema. Thermal or chemical burns may also result in airway edema. Late in hospitalization, contractures may limit neck mobility and mouth opening. Tracheostomy carries high morbidity and mortality in burn patients.

Aspiration Precautions   Routine.

Queries for Surgeon   Extent and sites of graft?

➤ **Anesthetic Considerations**
  1. **Preoperative Evaluation and Optimization**
     Routine history, physical examination, and laboratory studies. Pay special attention to associated underlying conditions (chronically debilitated patient with pressure sores or extensive burn patient).
  2. **Anesthetic Problems**
     a. Burn patient considerations
        (1) Airway
        (2) Respiratory (risk of pneumonia or ARDS) system
        (3) Cardiovascular system (extensive fluid requirements initial 48 hours; cardiac depression)
        (4) Poikilothermic state (in major burn patients, prevent temperature losses by keeping room temperature at 28° to 30° C, using fluid warmer and humidifier, and by covering exposed surfaces)
        (5) Metabolic (electrolyte, calcium disturbances) state
        (6) Endocrine (stress-related glucose intolerance) system
        (7) Hematologic (coagulopathy) system
        (8) Infection (pay exquisite attention to sterility with procedures)
        (9) Pharmacologically induced (succinylcholine) severe hyperkalemia occurs 2 to 3 days after burn
        (10) Increased nondepolarizing agent and analgesic requirements
     b. Monitoring. Routine ECG pads and BP cuff may be difficult to apply in extensive burn patients. Needle electrodes, BP cuff, and even IVs may need to be applied over burned areas.
     c. Blood loss can be surprisingly large with an apparently superficial procedure.
     d. Pain. Often excruciating after excision and grafting procedures.

Postoperative Pain Intensity Severe, particularly at donor site.

Postoperative Pain Control Local infiltration; parenteral or oral narcotics or both.

SUGGESTED READINGS

De Campo T, Aldrete JA. Anesthetic Management of the Severely Burned Patient. Intensive Care Med 7:55, 1981.

Lamb D. Anesthetic Considerations for Major Thermal Injury. Can Anesth Soc J 32:84, 1985.

CHAPTER 12

UROLOGIC
PROCEDURES

SURGICAL PROCEDURE   Extracorporeal Shock Wave Lithotripsy (ESWL)

Usually requires about 2000 to 4000 pulses synchronized with the electro-cardiogram (ECG). Newer generation lithotriptors may not be coupled to ECG. Lithotripsy with first generation lithotriptors is contraindicated in patients weighing more than 135 kg.

Objective   To fragment urinary calculi by extracorporeal shock wave application.

Position   If a ureteral stent is to be placed initially, patient is in lithotomy position.
1. *First generation lithotriptors.* The patient is immersed in water in a sitting position in a hydraulic lift (Fig. 5). Arms are left to float in the water. The head is on a head rest.
2. *Newer generation lithotriptors.* Do not require immersion in water. Patient is generally supine on table.

Exposure   There is no operative exposure. Stone localization is by x-ray control. Lithotripsy units are frequently at a distance from the main OR.

Incision   None.

Preoperative Studies   Routine.

Blood Bank Order   None.

Estimated Blood Loss   None.

Anesthetic Choices   General, regional (T4 level), or IV sedation. Equipment must be set up to carry out general anesthesia at all times. Standard anesthetic approach is IV sedation with newer generation lithotripsy machines because there is less pain with shocks. If patient is unable to cooperate, general anesthesia is preferred.

Invasive Monitoring   As indicated.

Airway Considerations   Standard or routine.

Aspiration Precautions   None unless general anesthesia is selected and patient is at risk of gastric reflux.

Estimated Surgical Time   Depends on number of shocks required and power of equipment. Average 1 to 2 hours.

➤ **Anesthetic Considerations**
  1. **Preoperative Considerations**
     Contraindications to ESWL are
     a. Pregnancy
     b. Aortic aneurysm
     c. Significant coagulation disorders
     d. Cardiac pacemaker
     e. Morbid obesity
  2. **Intraoperative Concerns and Goals**
     a. Radiation exposure to personnel.
     b. Positioning problems (logistics, injuries).
     c. Close observation of monitoring devices is required because of the considerable noise and physical distance from the patient.
     d. Immersion in water entails the following considerations:
        (1) Waterproof ECG pads required. BP cuff on arm immersed in water. Replace ECG pads frequently. Patient needs to be lifted from bath for ECG replacement.
        (2) Respiratory compromise due to elevation of diaphragm, decreased functional residual capacity, and increased atelectasis.
        (3) Immersion increases systemic vascular resistance and BP and decreases cardiac output. Patients with cardiac insufficiency may not tolerate ESWL.
     e. To keep the stone at the focal point of the lithotriptor (F_2 focus), minimize movement of patient.
     f. New generation lithotripsy machines do not require immersion in water. Treatment is on table. Anesthesia then consists of light analgesia (IV sedation).

Intraoperative Hazards
  1. Cardiac arrhythmias due to rapid changes in right heart filling pressures during transfer in and out of bath and to shock waves themselves eliciting arrhythmias (minimized with coupling of lithotriptor with ECG and with newer machines)
  2. Hyperthermia and hypothermia due to water immersion
  3. Perinephric hematoma
  4. Superficial skin bruising and occasionally bleeding
  5. Ureteral obstruction

Postoperative Pain Intensity   None, except with passage of stones or stone fragments.

Postoperative Pain Control   None.

SURGICAL PROCEDURE Kidney Transplantation

Healthy kidney is transplanted either from living related donor or cadaver donors. Procedure does not involve removal of nonfunctional kidneys in recipient.

Objective Transplantation of healthy kidney into patient with nonfunctioning kidneys.

Position Supine.

Exposure Nipples to pubis.

Incision Right or left lower quadrant. Donor kidney placed in iliac fossa in adults.

Blood Bank Order 2 units PRBCs.

Estimated Blood Loss 300 to 500 ml. Massive loss rare.

Preoperative Studies CBC, coagulation profile, electrolytes, CA^{2+}, PO_4, BUN, creatinine, glucose, ECG, CXR.

Anesthetic Choices General anesthesia with oral endotracheal tube (OETT); regional technique; or combined (general and regional) technique. Advantages of regional are less exposure to anesthetic drugs (not a major advantage) and avoidance of tracheal intubation. Coagulopathy is a contraindication to regional anesthesia.

Invasive Monitoring Foley; central venous catheter (CVC) and arterial line optional. CVC used for fluid hydration, to monitor central venous pressures and optimize renal hemodynamics, and for postoperative blood drawing and drug administration. Arterial line is not necessary in most patients unless BP is unstable.

Airway Considerations None.

Aspiration Precautions Often necessary because patient not NPO for previous 6 hours and because of possible gastroparesis due to chronic renal failure–related autonomic neuropathy.

➤ **Anesthetic Considerations**
  1. **Preoperative Evaluation**
     Based on history, physical examination, and laboratory studies; give special consideration to:
     a. Associated conditions in chronic renal failure: cardiovascular disease, hypertension, gastrointestinal abnormalities (including autonomic neuropathy with resultant gastroparesis), metabolic abnormalities (namely in K^+, Ca^{2+}, Mg^{2+}, PO_4), and hematologic abnormalities in hematocrit and platelet dysfunction.
     b. Polypharmacology including steroids and cardiovascular drugs.
     c. Dialysis-hemodialysis versus continuous ambulatory peritoneal dialysis (CAPD). Pay special attention to most recent hemodialysis run

and posthemodialysis laboratory studies and protect extremity with vascular access.

2. **Anesthetic Goals**
   a. Evaluate and optimize patient preoperatively.
   b. Aim for normal or above normal circulating blood volume and blood pressures during and after surgery.
   c. Pharmacologic considerations
      (1) Avoid drugs chiefly excreted by the kidneys, e.g., metacurine or even pancuronium.
      (2) Avoid nephrotoxic drugs, e.g., ethrane and aminoglycosides.
      (3) Avoid succinylcholine if K^+ >5.5 mEq/L.
   d. If using general anesthetic, aim for extubation immediately after surgery.
3. **Anesthetic Technique**
   a. Monitoring. After verifying patient identity and checking for most recent metabolic laboratory test results, place BP cuff and IV access in nonvascular access extremity. Nerve stimulator is useful because of altered pharmacokinetics of drugs. Invasive monitoring, if chosen, is usually placed after induction.
   b. Typical general anesthetic; preoxygenated, cricoid pressure and rapid-sequence induction with thiopental, succinylcholine, and fentanyl (3 to 5 µg/kg). Maintained on oxygen, N_2O, isoflurane, and atracurium. Regional may be used, although probably is not ideal because of extent of peritoneal dissection and retraction.
   c. Extubate immediately after surgery.
   d. Immunosuppressive drugs, antibiotics, and diuretics given during procedure.

Postoperative Management   Monitor urine output, CVC, BP, and chemistries.

Postoperative Pain Control   Optimally with epidural or PCA.

SURGICAL PROCEDURE   Nephrostomy Tube Placement

Objective   To drain kidney obstructed by stone or infections or by congenital ureteropelvic junction obstruction.

Position   Most often done percutaneously in genitourinary (GU) radiology area but can accompany pyeloplasty, usually in prone (Fig. 4) or lateral jackknife position (Fig. 2B).

Exposure   Iliac crest to nipple, flank, and posteriorly.

Incision   Usually percutaneous.

Blood Bank Order   T&S. Blood loss unusual but may necessitate open surgery.

Estimated Blood Loss   Less than 100 ml.

Preoperative Studies   HCT, electrolytes, BUN, creatinine.

Anesthetic Choices   General with endotracheal intubation; or regional (e.g., thoracic or lumbar epidural). Thoracic epidural anesthesia is effective and well tolerated. For example, 6 to 8 ml of 1.5% lidocaine through a T7–T10 epidural catheter suffices.

Invasive Monitoring   None.

Airway Considerations   Routine.

Aspiration Precautions   None unless an emergency procedure or patient is at risk of gastric reflux.

Estimated Surgical Time   2 hours.

➤ **Anesthetic Considerations**
1. **Preoperative Considerations**
   Associated medical conditions, e.g., renal failure.
2. **Intraoperative Considerations**
   Positioning the patient in the lateral decubitus position with elevation of the kidney bar may produce venous pooling or mechanical obstruction of venous return.

Intraoperative Hazards
1. Bacteremia and consequent hemodynamic instability with manipulation of obstructed kidney
2. Renal trauma
3. Bleeding
4. Pneumothorax

Postoperative Pain Intensity   Mild to moderate.

Postoperative Pain Control   Parenteral analgesics.

Postoperative Tests   HCT, CXR to rule out pneumothorax.

SURGICAL PROCEDURE   Open Prostatectomy

Includes suprapubic (transvesical), retropubic, and perineal approaches as opposed to transurethral approach.

Objective   To remove benign adenoma or the entire prostate with the seminal vesicles and vas deferens (for cancer). Most often indicated for large prostates (>60 g) that are too difficult to resect transurethrally.

Position   Exaggerated lithotomy (Fig. 3) or lithotomy with Trendelenburg.

Exposure   Perineal—perineum and genitalia. The rectum is draped out of field with plastic tape or sutured skin towel. Retropubic and suprapubic—symphysis to genitalia.

Incision   Perineal—a curvilinear perineal incision that extends from the two ischiorectal fossae. Retropubic and suprapubic—a suprapubic incision.

Preoperative Studies   Routine.

Blood Bank Order   T&C 2 units PRBCs.

Estimated Blood Loss   Approximately 500 ml.

Anesthetic Choices   General, epidural, spinal. Given the position, there may be restriction of thoracic excursion with resultant hypoxemia.

Invasive Monitoring   None.

Airway Considerations   Routine.

Aspiration Precautions   Standard.

Estimated Surgical Time   2 to 3 hours.

➤ **Anesthetic Considerations**
1. **Preoperative Considerations**
   Often an elderly patient population, some with associated medical problems.
2. **Anesthetic Considerations**
   a. Special attention to positioning. Shoulder braces may produce brachial plexus injury.
   b. Selection of patients for regional. Positioning and cooperation a problem for many.
   c. Pulmonary compromise with lithotomy or Trendelenburg positioning.
   d. Potential for major blood loss and large third space losses, although not as much as for radical prostatectomy.

Intraoperative Hazards
1. Rectal injury may require colostomy.
2. Sores at pressure points.

Postoperative Pain Intensity   Moderate.

Postoperative Pain Control   PCA, routine.

SURGICAL PROCEDURE   Percutaneous Lithotripsy

Involves removal of stones through a percutaneous puncture site; insertion of in-dwelling stents; ultrasonic lithotripsy.

Objective   Removal of stone fragments or foreign bodies or stricture release.

Position   Prone on the C-arm table (Fig. 4*A*).

Exposure   Iliac crest to nipple, flank, and posteriorly.

Incision   The procedure is done through a percutaneous site, which usually is prepared beforehand. On occasion, a percutaneous puncture may be done in the operating room under ultrasound control.

Preoperative Studies   Renal function, electrolytes, HCT, coagulation profile.

Blood Bank Order   T&S.

Estimated Blood Loss   Insignificant unless vessel injury occurs.

Anesthetic Choices   General, regional (T4 level), or IV sedation and local. Paraplegics (relatively high incidence of nephrolithiasis) with level of spinal cord injury above T7 usually require general anesthesia or regional for prevention or control of autonomic hyperreflexia.

Invasive Monitoring   Foley.

Airway Considerations   Oral endotracheal tube (OETT) if general anesthesia is used.

Aspiration Precautions   Not unless an emergency procedure or patient is at risk of gastric reflux.

Estimated Surgical Time   Variable, although often less than 1 hour.

Queries to Surgeon   Projected duration of procedure?

➤ **Anesthetic Considerations**
1. **Preoperative Considerations**
   a. Stringent criteria for selection of patients for local with IV sedation: Procedure is painful and often prolonged. Prone positioning increases respiratory and hemodynamic compromise and precludes converting local anesthetic technique to general anesthesia.
   b. Associated medical problems include renal compromise and paraplegia.
2. **Intraoperative Considerations**
   a. With prone positioning, pay special attention to pressure points and eyes.
   b. Extensive use of fluoroscopy.

Intraoperative Hazards
1. Bleeding
2. Respiratory compromise
3. Hemodynamic compromise
4. Pneumothorax
5. Agitation
6. Extubation a risk when patient is being log rolled into position and in prone position

Postoperative Problems
1. Pneumothorax
2. Bleeding

Postoperative Pain Intensity   Mild to moderate.

Postoperative Pain Control   Routine; epidural and PCA.

Postoperative Tests   HCT, CXR.

SURGICAL PROCEDURE   Radical Cystectomy

Indicated for papillomatosis and for high-grade invasive tumors. Most vesical neoplasms are transitional cell type. Multifocal and recurrent tumors are common. Gross hematuria is most common presenting symptom. Diagnosis is confirmed by cystoscopy and biopsy.

Objective   Removal in the male of bladder, prostate, seminal vesicles, and ampulla of the vas deferens, along with the peritoneal covering of these structures and the lymph nodes of the true pelvis. In women the bladder, the uterus, tubes and ovaries, and the anterior vaginal wall are removed. Urinary diversion through an ileal or colonic conduit is accomplished. Gastrostomy is often performed. An appendectomy is included.

Position   Trendelenburg, supine. Use intermittent pressure boots for DVT prevention.

Exposure   Nipples to pubis.

Incision   Left paramedian from symphysis through the midhypochondrium. Occasionally transverse incision from iliac spine to iliac spine.

Preoperative Studies   Renal function, HCT, coagulation profile, electrolytes, glucose, LFTs, ECG, CXR.

Blood Bank Order   T&C 4 units PRBCs. Keep 2 units available throughout procedure.

Estimated Blood Loss   May be more than 1000 ml.

Anesthetic Choices   General or combined general and epidural.

Invasive Monitoring   Arterial line and central venous catheter useful because of large fluid shifts and possible appreciable blood loss. Unable to monitor urine output.

Airway Considerations   Routine.

Aspiration Precautions   None unless an emergency procedure or patient is at risk of gastric reflux.

Estimated Surgical Time   5 to 8 hours.

➤ **Anesthetic Considerations**
1. **Preoperative Considerations**
   a. Associated medical conditions
   b. Often an elderly or debilitated population
2. **Intraoperative Considerations**
   a. Potential for significant blood and fluid losses. Before induction, verify availability of blood and that adequate large-bore IV access and monitoring equipment is on hand.
   b. Factors cited above and length of procedure increase risk of hypothermia.
   c. Vagal reaction possible with manipulation and traction of bowel.
   d. Because of bowel distension, avoid giving >50% N_2O or even any N_2O.
   e. In patients who have received radiation therapy, surgical dissection may be more difficult and bloody.
   f. Aim to extubate immediately at end of procedure.
   g. Postoperative analgesia considerations.

Intraoperative Hazards
1. Prolonged surgery
2. Unable to assess urine output
3. Large third space losses
4. Major blood loss potential
5. Hypothermia

Postoperative Problems
1. Coagulopathy
2. Bleeding
3. Hypovolemia
4. Pulmonary embolus
5. Nonanion gap metabolic acidosis and hypokalemia from urinary diversion
6. Appreciable third space losses continuing

Postoperative Pain Intensity   Severe.

Postoperative Pain Control   Epidural, PCA, Routine parenteral.

Postoperative Tests   CXR, ECG, HCT, coagulation profile, electrolytes, urine output.

SURGICAL PROCEDURE   Radical Nephrectomy

Indicated for malignant renal tumors. Mostly adenocarcinoma: a common malignant neoplasm arising from renal tubular cells. Tends to invade renal vein and inferior vena cava (IVC). Right-sided neoplasms more likely to involve IVC than left-sided tumors are. Classic triad of renal cell carcinoma—mass, pain, and hematuria—is seen in less than half the patients. Painless hematuria most common presentation. Diagnosis usually confirmed by intravenous pyelogram (IVP) or CT scan or both.

Objective   Removal of kidney encased in perirenal fat, fascia, and local lymph nodes. Early mobilization and ligation of renal vessels minimizes venous tumor spread and blood loss.

Position Lateral (Fig. 2), with nephrectomy side up, arms extended and supported, downside brachial plexus protected, downside knee bent after being aligned with the superior anterior iliac crest over the table break. Variations on this position, especially to a ¾ position with the patient turned and fixed more anteriorly, may be used if a thoracolumbar or thoracoabdominal incision is planned.

Exposure Depends on operative approach.

Incision The operative approach may be through the flank, abdomen, or chest.

Preoperative Studies Renal function, HCT, coagulation profile, electrolytes, CXR. Renal scan to determine functioning of contralateral kidney; evaluation of extension of tumor for carcinoma (e.g., CT scan, IVC venogram).

Blood Bank Order T&C 4 units PRBCs.

Estimated Blood Loss 500 ml.

Anesthetic Choices General; epidural optional.

Invasive Monitoring Central venous catheter; arterial line useful but not essential.

Airway Considerations Standard.

Aspiration Precautions There may be ileus, increased abdominal pressure, or impressive preoperative use of narcotics. If so, consider the patient an aspiration precaution on induction.

Queries for Surgeon
1. Is the superior mesenteric artery involved? (Blood supply to colon may be compromised. If so, possible colonic resection.)
2. Is there tumor high in the vena cava? (If so, prepare for possible cardiopulmonary bypass and deep hypothermic circulatory arrest beforehand.)

Estimated Surgical Time 2 to 4 hours.

▶ **Anesthetic Considerations**
1. **Preoperative Considerations**
    a. Cancer patient with higher risk of other medical problems.
    b. Accurate delineation of tumor extension (vascular, bowel).
    c. Preoperative chemotherapy or radiation therapy.
2. **Intraoperative Concerns**
    a. Positioning.
    b. Potential for massive hemorrhage.
    c. Large third space fluid requirements.
    d. Hypothermia.
    e. Paralysis for adequate surgical exposure.

    f. Pharmacologic protection of contralateral kidney (e.g., mannitol, renal-dose dopamine).
    g. Hemodynamic compromise due to IVC clamping (if necessary).
    h. Infected kidney causes bacteremia during surgical manipulation.
    i. High IVC and right atrial extension of tumor may require cardiopulmonary bypass with circulatory arrest.
    j. Postoperative analgesic considerations.

Postoperative Problems
1. Pneumothorax in extrapleural incisions
2. Pain
3. Atelectasis
4. Bleeding
5. Hypoxemia
6. Oliguria
7. Hypothermia
8. Continued appreciable third space losses

Postoperative Pain Intensity   Severe.

Postoperative Pain Control   Epidural, PCA, or routine parenteral.

Postoperative Tests   CXR, HCT, ABGs, urine output.

SURGICAL PROCEDURE Radical Retropubic Prostatectomy

Indicated for cancer of the prostate.

Objective   Removal of pelvic nodes and complete removal of the prostate, seminal vesicles, and ampulla of the vas deferens.

Position   Trendelenburg: greater trochanters at the table break. Intent is to achieve maximal distance between the symphysis and the umbilicus.

Exposure   Symphysis to umbilicus. The penis is prepared and draped out of the field with an indwelling catheter.

Incision   Above umbilicus with transperitoneal approach or below umbilicus with extraperitoneal approach. Sometimes transverse incision from iliac spine to iliac spine with midline bowing.

Preoperative Studies   HCT, coagulation profile, electrolytes, BUN, creatinine, glucose, ECG. Metastatic workup includes CXR, alkaline phosphatase, PSA (prostatic specific antigen), LFTs, CA^{2+}, PO_4.

Blood Bank Order   T&C 4 units PRBCs; keep 2 ahead.

Estimated Blood Loss   Approximately 1000 ml; may be much more.

Anesthetic Choices   General; regional optional. Postoperative epidural narcotic analgesia useful.

Invasive Monitoring   Arterial line, central venous catheter useful because of potential for significant blood and third space losses, especially in elderly patient population.

Airway Considerations   Routine.

Aspiration Precautions   None unless an emergency procedure or patient is at risk of gastric reflux.

➤ **Anesthetic Considerations**
1. **Preoperative Considerations**
   Generally an elderly patient population with associated medical problems.
2. **Anesthetic Concerns and Goals**
   a. Procedure approached as a major abdominal case.
   b. Estimated blood loss is large.
   c. Large third space losses.
   d. Potential for hypothermia, coagulopathy or disseminated intravascular coagulation, and bacteremia.
   e. Large-bore IV access.
   f. Pay special attention to positioning because procedure is lengthy.
   g. Hypotension due to poor vascular tone or positioning.
   h. Paralysis for better surgical exposure.

Intraoperative Hazards
1. Massive bleeding (not uncommon with this procedure)
2. Hypovolemia
3. Hypothermia
4. Coagulopathy
5. Rectal injury

Estimated Surgical Time   3 to 5 hours.

Postoperative Management   PACU or ICU. Overnight monitoring in ICU or PACU useful for fluid management and monitoring for postoperative complications (e.g., hemodynamics, blood loss, cardiac risk).

Postoperative Pain Intensity   Moderate.

Postoperative Pain Control   Epidural, PCA, routine.

Postoperative Tests   HCT, coagulation profile, ECG.

SURGICAL PROCEDURE   Transurethral Resection of Prostate

Transurethral prostatectomy (TURP) is indicated for benign prostatic hypertrophy causing major urinary obstruction. Characterized by difficulty voiding, frequency, and nocturia. Approach also employed for relief of urinary obstruction in surgically incurable carcinoma of the prostate. The procedure is performed by application of a high-frequency current to a wire loop. To prevent diffusion of the current, glycine is used as a continuous irrigant.

Objective   Relief of urinary obstruction.

Position   Lithotomy.

Exposure   Genitalia; a special drape covers the perineal area. One perforation in drape allows the penis to be reached.

Incision   None unless urologist adds bilateral vasectomy.

Preoperative Studies   CBC, coagulation profile, electrolytes, BUN, creatinine, glucose, ECG; CXR optional.

Blood Bank Order   T&S.

Estimated Blood Loss   Depends on extent of procedure; approximately 300 ml.

Anesthetic Choices   General, spinal, epidural. Spinal is preferred technique because it permits monitoring of mental status for hyponatremia.

Invasive Monitoring   None.

Airway Considerations   Routine.

Aspiration Precautions   None unless an emergency procedure or patient is at risk of gastric reflux.

Queries for Surgeon   Size of gland? (Large gland [>60 g] requires retropubic approach.) Duration of procedure? (Tailor regional anesthetic dose.)

Estimated Surgical Time   Usually 1 to 1½ hours.

▶ **Anesthetic Considerations**
 1. **Preoperative Considerations**
    Generally an elderly patient population with decreased physiologic reserve and often a multitude of medical problems.
 2. **Anesthetic Concerns**
    a. TURP syndrome, caused by irrigant fluid absorption, results in fluid overload, glycine toxicity (can produce retinal blindness or hyperammonia-related encephalopathy), hyponatremia (severity related to rapidity of sodium concentration changes and absolute concentration; symptoms generally not seen until sodium concentration <120 mEq/L), coagulopathy, bacteremia or sepsis and hypothermia.
    b. Potential for bladder perforation.
    c. Judicious use of sedation in the elderly patient at risk of benzodiazepine-induced agitation.
    d. Associated medical problems in a generally elderly population.
    e. Hypovolemia due to blood loss that may range from minimal to greater than 2000 ml.
    f. Fluid absorption related to surgical skill, size of prostate, height of

irrigant fluid, duration of procedure. Average fluid absorption approximately 2 L.

Intraoperative Hazards
1. Pulmonary edema.
2. Mental status changes with consequent agitation or obtundation due to hyponatremia are associated with the TURP syndrome.
3. Seizures.
4. Septic hemodynamics due to manipulation of infected prostate.
5. Disseminated intravascular coagulation from prostatic fibrinolytic substances.
6. Regional-related complications, e.g., hypotension from high spinal.
7. Prostatic capsule or bladder perforation resulting in acute abdomen.

Treatment of hyponatremia is guided by symptoms and absolute values. Symptomatic patients with Na^+ concentration <120 mEq/L should be promptly treated with diuretics and 0.9% to 3% NaCl. Prostatic capsule perforation requires drainage by extravesicular approach or cystotomy.

Postoperative Problems
1. Hyponatremia-induced cerebral edema, seizures, coma, or central pontine myelinolysis (Central pontine myelinolysis is pontine demyelination related to hyponatremia and to the rapidity of sodium changes. Characterized by severe neurologic symptoms, coma, and death.)
2. Manifestations of bladder rupture with signs of acute abdomen
3. Bleeding
4. Foley catheter obstruction

Postoperative Pain Intensity   Moderate, especially bladder discomfort.

Postoperative Pain Control   Routine.

Postoperative Tests Na^+ concentration, coagulation profile, HCT; ECG if indicated.

SUGGESTED READINGS
Bready LL. Kidney Transplantation. In Anesthesiology Clinics of North America. Philadelphia: W.B. Saunders, Vol #7, Sept 1989.

Liu WS, Wong KC. Anesthesia for Genitourinary Surgery. In Barash P (ed), Clinical Anesthesia. London: J.B. Lippincott, 1992.

Weber W, Peter K, Negri L, Schelling G. Anesthesia for ESWL. In Nunn JF (ed), General Anesthesia. London: Buttersworth, 1989.

APPENDIX I

Common Surgical Positions

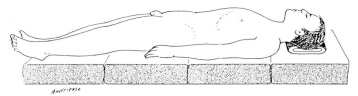

Figure 1. The traditional supine position.

CONSIDERATIONS

1. Ensure preparation of OR table before patient's arrival, e.g., warming blanket.
2. Pay special attention to potential pressure points: face from mask, mask strap, or endotracheal tube (ETT); ulnar nerve injury from pressure posterior to medial condyle (elbow pads may prevent ulnar nerve injury); radial nerve injury from pressure in upper arm where nerve spirals around humerus (e.g., by metal screen holder); crossed legs.
3. Protect eyes from corneal abrasions and from drying by taping eyes shut with or without eye lubricant. (Check patients for contact lenses, especially trauma patients brought in unconscious.)
4. Beware of head extension or flexion movement resulting in ETT displacement (i.e., extubation or endobronchial intubation).
5. Change scalp resting points in prolonged procedures to avoid creation of bald spot. Ensure grounding and avoid patient's contact with metal surfaces.
6. Avoid > 90-degree arm abduction to prevent brachial plexus injury.
7. Ensure access to an upper extremity in the event of need for additional IV access, arterial line, twitch monitors, repositioning of BP cuff, or SaO_2 monitor.
8. Ensure proper functioning of IV and arterial lines after final positioning.
9. Provide lumbar support in the form of an inflatable wedge to help prevent postoperative backache.
10. Pneumatic compression boots useful for prolonged procedures in DVT prophylaxis.
11. Place belt around thighs of agitated patient to prevent his falling off OR table.

CONSIDERATIONS
1. Anesthesia induced while patient is in supine position.
2. Use care in log rolling patient.
3. Place IV in uppermost arm and central venous catheter in uppermost neck for ease of access.
4. Ensure proper head support to prevent brachial plexus stretching and injury, and that ear is not trapped or folded onto itself.
5. Avoid pressure from edge of upper arm support.
6. Use axillary roll in attempt to prevent lower arm brachial plexus injury.
7. Flex lower leg at knee and hip.
8. Protect bony prominences with pillows, e.g., between legs.
9. Table flexed for greater thoracic or flank exposure.

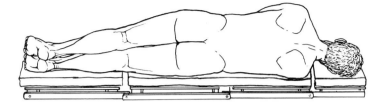

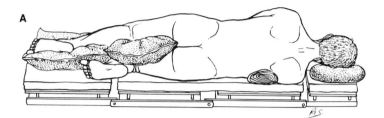

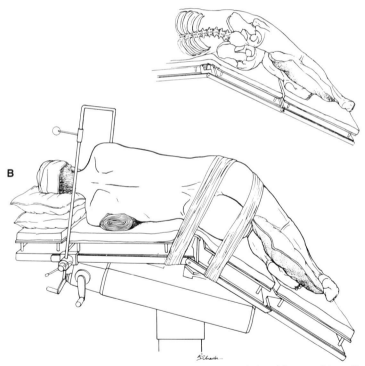

Figure 2. Lateral position. *A,* Standard right lateral decubitus position. *B,* Lateral jackknife position; table flexion is at level of iliac crest. In the semiprone position (not shown), downside arm is alongside and behind torso to avoid axillary compression. Indications include renal, extraperitoneal, thoracic, orthopedic, neurosurgical (unflexed table) procedures.

Illustration from Martin JT. Positioning in Anesthesia and Surgery, ed 2. Philadelphia: W.B. Saunders, 1987.

CONSIDERATIONS

1. Lower extremity at risk of pressure points and multiple neurologic injuries. Namely, common perineal nerve from stirrup compression at the head of the fibula; saphenous nerve from compression at the medial tibial condyle; femoral nerve injury due to kinking under the inguinal ligament associated with flexion and abduction of thighs. Other nerve injuries include sciatic and obturator nerves and posterior tibial nerve at the popliteal fossa.
2. Increased perineal exposure can be provided by pad under sacrum.
3. Use of shoulder supports avoided because of documented association with brachial plexus injury.
4. Raise legs together to avoid sprain injuries at level of pelvis and hips.
5. Always watch that the patient's fingers are not caught in the table when elevating leg section.

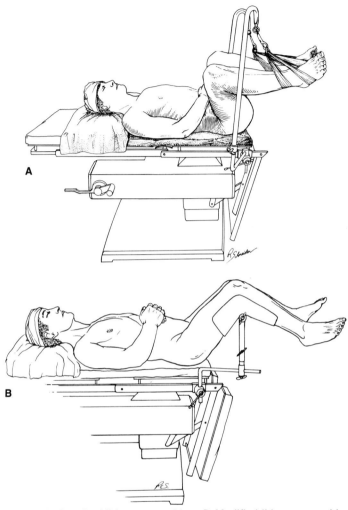

Figure 3. *A,* Standard lithotomy position. *B,* Modified lithotomy position. A variation is the lithotomy-Trendelenburg position (not shown) used in pelvic procedures. Indications include anal procedures (e.g., hemorrhoidectomy), abdominoperineal procedures (e.g., colorectal), and laparoscopy for gynecologic or urologic procedures.

Illustration from Martin JT. Positioning in Anesthesia and Surgery, ed 2. Philadelphia: W.B. Saunders, 1987.

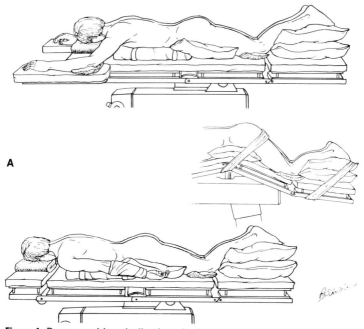

A

Figure 4. Prone position. Indications include surgery on posterior aspect of body, e.g., plastic, spinal axis and neurosurgical procedures. There are various modifications in the prone position and various frame setups. Examples: *A,* Classic prone position. *B,* Kneeling position with hip and knees flexed at 90 degrees for lumbosacral surgery. *C,* Prone jackknife for anorectal or pilonidal cyst procedures.

Illustration from Martin JT. Positioning in Anesthesia and Surgery, ed 2. Philadelphia: W.B. Saunders Co., 1987. **B** Redrawn with permission of Orthopedic Systems, Inc., Hayward, California.

CONSIDERATIONS

1. Position with highest risk for injuries.
2. Allow abdomen to be free, as abdominal pressure causes IVC obstruction, venous back-pressure, and consequently more blood loss at the operative site as well as impaired ventilation. Epigastric pressure causes liver sinusoidal congestion, whereas groin pressure compresses the neurovascular bundle.
3. Protect those areas at risk for compression injuries: eyes, nose, breasts, male genitalia, and bony prominences such as the anterior superior iliac spines, the knees, and toes. Thus, tape eyes shut after induction and protect eyes and nose from pressure throughout the procedure. Check under patient's body that the breasts and genitalia are not malpositioned and place pillows under patient's lower legs to relieve pressure on toes.
4. Keep head in neutral position and avoid hyperextension of the neck.
5. Arms may be kept either alongside the patient or above the head. Extension of the arms on arm boards has been shown to result in neurologic compromise.

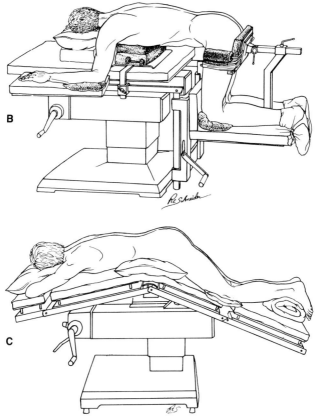

Figure 4–cont'd. For legend, see opposite page.

6. Ensure secure fixation of endotracheal tube because of risk of extubation in prone position. Also pay special attention to IVs and central venous catheters.
7. Induction and intubation may be performed with the patient in the supine position on his own bed or on the OR table.
8. Turning patient into prone position requires careful planning, clear understanding by all those involved, controlled movement, disconnecting patient from ventilator and all monitors, and allowing sufficient slack in IV and transducer lines. Pay very careful attention to the head and the lower arm during lifting and log rolling of patient. Verify that ventilator and monitor are reconnected; confirm bilateral breath sounds and $ETCO_2$, and check that all pressure points discussed above are protected.
9. Alternatively for increased safety, patients can be intubated and then positioned awake (if at all possible with the airway well topicalized and patient well sedated).

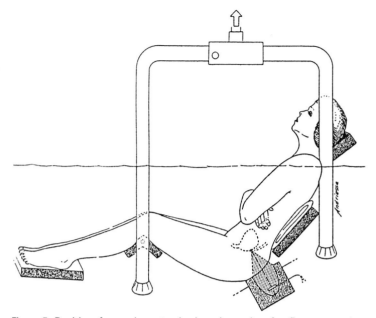

Figure 5. Position for underwater body submersion for first generation extracorporeal shock wave lithotripsy (ESWL). See Chapter 12, ESWL discussion, for considerations.

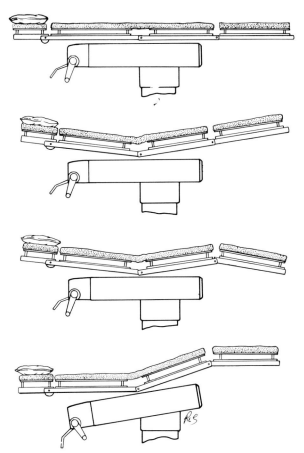

Figure 6. Lawn chair position. Adds to patient's comfort, especially in prolonged procedures in which regional anesthetic is used.

Illustrations from Martin JT. Positioning in Anesthesia and Surgery, ed 2. Philadelphia: W.B. Saunders, 1987.

CONSIDERATIONS

1. Flexion of knees and hips places joints in more anatomically neutral position.
2. Better distribution of dorsal surface.
3. Slight upright posture facilitates breathing.

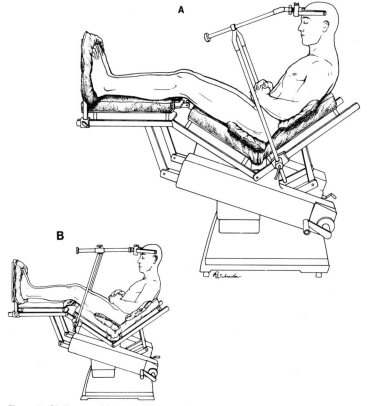

Figure 7. Sitting position used in craniotomies and cervical laminectomies with pin-type head holders (e.g., Mayfield skull clamp). This is a variation of the lawn chair position shown in Figure 6.

Illustration from Martin JT. Positioning in Anesthesia and Surgery, ed 2. Philadelphia: W.B. Saunders Co., 1987.

COMMONLY USED MEDICAL ABBREVIATIONS

ABCs	Airway, breathing, circulation
ABGs	Arterial blood gases
ACT	Activated clotting time
ALT	Alanine aminotransferase
ASA	American Society of Anesthesiologists
AST	Aspartate aminotransferase
ATN	Acute tubular necrosis
AV	Atrioventricular
BP	Blood pressure
BUN	Blood urea nitrogen
CABG	Coronary artery bypass graft
CAD	Coronary artery disease
CAPD	Continuous ambulatory peritoneal dialysis
CAVH	Continuous arteriovenous hemofiltration
CHF	Congestive heart failure
CNS	Central nervous system
CO	Cardiac output
Coagulation profile	Prothrombin time, partial thromboplastin time, platelets, fibrinogen; disseminated intravascular coagulation workup as indicated
COPD	Chronic obstructive pulmonary disease
CPAP	Continuous positive airway pressure
CPB	Cardiopulmonary bypass
CPK	Creatine phosphokinase
CSF	Cerebrospinal fluid
CT	Computed tomography
CVC	Central venous catheter
CVP	Central venous pressure
CXR	Chest x-ray examination
DIC	Disseminated intravascular coagulation
DLETT	Double-lumen endotracheal tube
DM	Diabetes mellitus
DVT	Deep venous thrombosis
$D_{2.5}W$	2.5% dextrose in water
D_5W	5% dextrose in water
$D_{10}W$	10% dextrose in water
ECG	Electrocardiogram
ER	Emergency room
$ETCO_2$	Partial pressure end-tidal CO_2
ETI	Endotracheal intubation
ETT	Endotracheal tube
FDP	Fibrin degradation products
FEV	Forced expiratory volume
FEV_1	Forced expiratory volume in 1 second

221

FHR	Fetal heart rate	NSAID	Nonsteroidal antiin-flammatory drug
FFP	Fresh-frozen plasma		
FIO_2	Fraction of inspired oxygen	OETI	Oral endotracheal intu-bation
Foley	Foley urinary catheter	OETT	Oral endotracheal tube
FRC	Functional residual ca-pacity	OR	Operating room
		PAC	Pulmonary artery cathe-ter or Swan-Ganz cathe-ter
GGT	Gamma glutamyl trans-ferase		
GI	Gastrointestinal	PIP	Peak inspiratory pres-sure
GU	Genitourinary		
Hb	Hemoglobin	PO	By mouth
HCT	Hematocrit	PACU	Postanesthesia care unit or recovery room
HR	Heart rate		
IABP	Intraaortic balloon pump	PCA	Patient-controlled anal-gesia
IAP	Intraabdominal pres-sure	PEEP	Positive end expiratory pressure
ICP	Intracranial pressure	PEG	Percutaneous endo-scopic gastrostomy
ICU	Intensive care unit		
ID	Identification; inner di-ameter	PFTs	Pulmonary function tests
IHSS	Idiopathic hypertrophic subaortic stenosis	PICU	Pediatric intensive care unit
IM	Intramuscular	PRBCs	Packed red blood cells
IV	Intravenous	PT	Prothrombin time
IVC	Inferior vena cava	PTT	Partial thromboplastin time
IVP	Intravenous pyelogram		
LBBB	Left bundle branch block	PUD	Peptic ulcer disease
		RBC	Red blood cell
LDH	Lactate dehydrogenase	RUQ	Right upper quadrant
LFTs	Liver function tests	RV	Residual volume
LVAD	Left ventricular assist device	s	Second
		SAH	Subarachnoid hemor-rhage
LVEF	Left ventricular ejection fraction		
		SIRS	Systemic inflammatory response syndrome
MAC	Minimum alveolar con-centration		
		SSEP	Somatosensory evoked potential
MI	Myocardial infarction		
MODS	Multiple organ dysfunc-tion syndrome	SVC	Superior vena cava
		SVR	Systemic vascular resis-tance
MRI	Magnetic resonance im-aging		
		SVT	Supraventricular tachy-cardia
MUGA	Multiple unit gated ac-quisition scan		
		T&A	Tonsillectomy and ade-noidectomy
MVV	Maximum voluntary ventilation		
		T&C	Type and crossmatch
NGT	Nasogastric tube	T&S	Type and screen
NICU	Neonatal intensive care unit	TEE	Transesophageal echo-cardiography
NPO	Nothing by mouth	TEF	Tracheoesophageal fis-tula
NS	Normal saline		

TFC	Thompson-Friedenrich cryptantigen
TLC	Total lung capacity
TOF	Train-of-four
TPN	Total parenteral nutrition
TT	Thrombin time
TURP	Transurethral prostatectomy
UGI	Upper gastrointestinal
VAE	Venous air embolus
VATER	Vertebral abnormalities, imperforate Anus, Tracheo-Esophageal fistula, Radial aplasia or Renal abnormalities
$\dot{V}/\dot{Q}$	Ventilation-perfusion ratio
V_T	Tidal volume

INDEX